RYAN HUNT

Intermittent Fasting

The Spartan Approach to Diet, Fat Loss, and Health

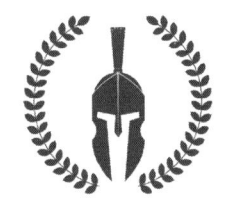

Copyright © 2018 by Ryan Hunt

All rights reserved. No part of this publication may be reproduced, stored or transmitted in any form or by any means, electronic, mechanical, photocopying, recording, scanning, or otherwise without written permission from the publisher. It is illegal to copy this book, post it to a website, or distribute it by any other means without permission.

Ryan Hunt has no responsibility for the persistence or accuracy of URLs for external or third-party Internet Websites referred to in this publication and does not guarantee that any content on such Websites is, or will remain, accurate or appropriate.

First edition

This book was professionally typeset on Reedsy.
Find out more at reedsy.com

Contents

Introduction	iv
The History of Fasting	1
The Story Behind Intermittent Fasting	14
Misunderstandings about Intermittent Fasting	24
Why Intermittent Fasting Works?	38
The Benefits of Intermittent Fasting	51
Can You Build Muscle with Intermittent Fasting?	62
What Are the Effects of Intermittent Fasting	72
An Intermittent Fasting Plan: A Practical Approach	83
What About Keto and Intermittent Fasting Combined?	108
Intermittent Fasting and Supplements	117
Tricks and Tips	131
Creating a Spartan Lifestyle of Intermittent Fasting	145
Conclusion	150
Disclaimer	152

Introduction

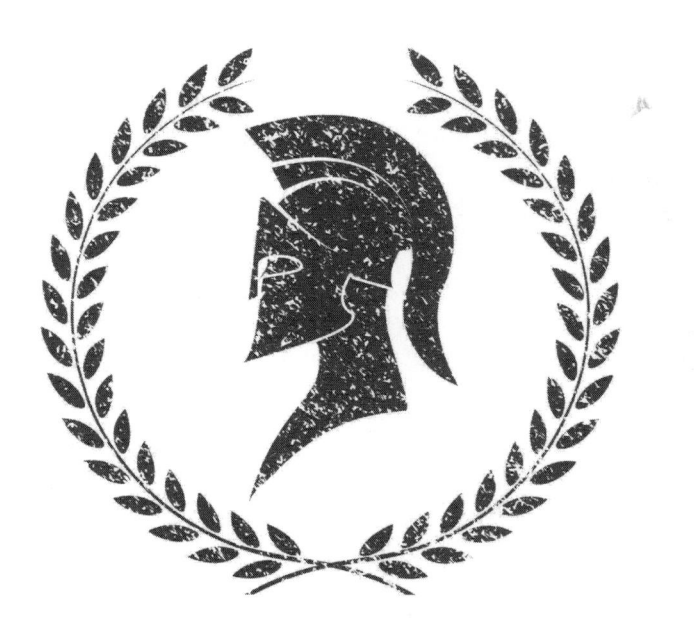

This book is your comprehensive beginner's guide on how you can start your journey towards a healthier and longer life through the ancient practice of intermittent fasting.

There are many forms of Intermittent Fasting - each with its own eating rules, recommended meals, and mindset. In this book, you will learn about the Spartan approach, which calls for the warrior within yourself.

You are probably aware of the Spartans thanks to the movie adaptation of the epic graphic novel 300. Aside from the godly physique of the army led by King Leonidas, the small band of warriors was noted for their never-give-up attitude and unbelievable courage.

But who were the Spartans and what is their connection with a diet regimen such as intermittent fasting?

Spartans refer to the citizens of Sparta - a major city-state in Ancient Greece. This warrior society reached their height of power after they defeated Athens, which is another major city-state in the Peloponnesian War (431 to 404 B.C). While Athens was noted for its democracy, the culture of its rival state Sparta was focused on the military service and loyalty to the state.

Spartan culture and practices were considered brutal even to the standards of the Ancient world when wars and strife were very common. In fact, Spartans were quite extreme that they had to start proving their fitness even as babies.

In the Ancient world, infanticide was common. However, in Sparta, this practice was sanctioned by the state. According to the historian Plutarch, newly born babies were required to be presented before a council for examining physical defects. Those who were not up to the standards of the warrior society were not allowed to live. Usually, these ill-fated babies were left on hillsides to die or sometimes to be rescued by strangers.

But this examination was only the start of succeeding harsh tests. The infants who passed the standards were regularly tested by their constitutions by bathing in wine rather than water. Parents were also required by the state not to take care of their children when they cried. Young Spartans were also commanded not to fear solitude or darkness.

When young boys reached the age of 7, they were commanded by the state to begin their training through a system known as agoge. This is an extreme regimen created to mold the young boys into warriors. The children were separated from their families and forced to live in barracks where they learned athletics, hunting, stealth, warfare, and scholastics.

By age 12, the young military trainees were only given a red cloak for their clothes and were required to sleep outside the barracks. As preparation in the field, they were forced to scavenge and steal food, and if they were caught, they were flogged.

While military service was only required for men, Spartan girls also underwent rigorous training. In Sparta, women were expected to bear children so that the population will be kept and ensure the continuity of the society. Young girls were allowed to live with their parents, but they had to train hard and learn discus throwing and javelin, which were believed to make them strong mothers. They were also trained in warfare in case the city was attacked by invaders and extra hands were needed for defense.

There were more harsh practices that the Spartans experienced. The stories and historical accounts inspired modern warfare. But what is the connection of this extreme regimen with intermittent fasting?

From the moment they were born, Spartans were subjected to stress, which is partly at the core of intermittent fasting. Later, you will learn why stress is crucial for living a healthier and longer life.

At age 21, Spartan men were expected to complete the primary stage of their training. Those who passed were elected to the military-style mess known as *syssitia* where citizens can gather to partake in a meal. But this was not a feast. The rations were doled out and the state managed the distribution of food. As such, Spartans were known for this proper diet and physical fitness. Overweight citizens were ostracized and generally loathed by the public.

Spartans were wine drinkers, but they were not alcoholics. The state discourages drunkenness and wild revelry. Children were cautioned against drunkenness, and in some instances, they would even force slaves to be drunk to show young Spartans the damaging effects of too much alcohol.

Willpower. Resolve. Courage. Moderation.

These are the strong values that Spartans embodied that made them effective as a warrior society. They were feared in the Ancient world and they won their battles.

Similarly, you can win your way towards health and wellness if you become a Spartan.

Of course, not literally. You don't need to undergo such harsh military training. Rather, you need to use the discipline and the mindset of the Spartans so you can reach your health goals through intermittent fasting.

Intermittent fasting has been making some buzz in the health world and many celebrities and athletes now claim that this regimen is part of their lifestyle. While intermittent fasting can be effective, it still requires dedication and discipline so you can see ultimate results.

Hopefully, this book will help you explore the wonderful benefits of intermittent fasting - its downsides, scientific basis, recommended meals, and many more.

Thank you for reading this book and I hope you enjoy!

1

The History of Fasting

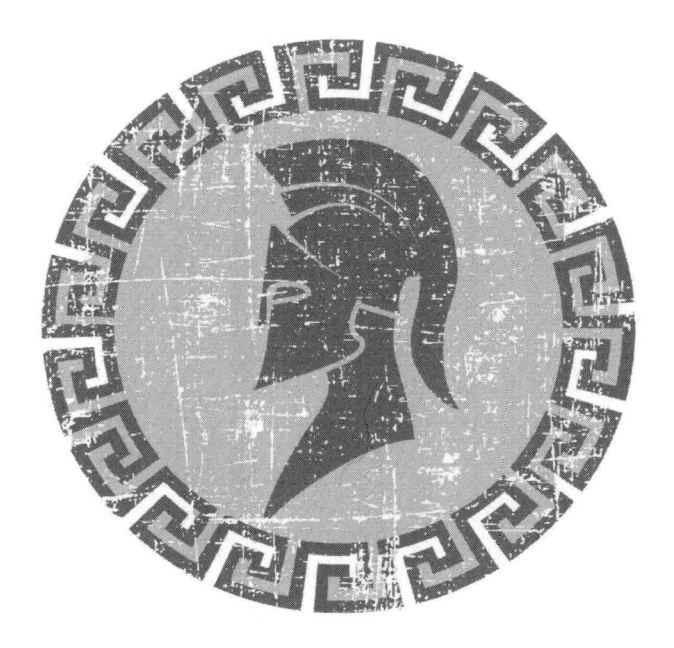

Fasting is an ancient practice that has been used by many civilizations not only for religious practices but also for its medicinal and wellness benefits.

There is no definitive beginning for the history of fasting because it is not logical to think that our ancestors did not practice fasting. Think about it. Early humans didn't have the abundance of food that we now enjoy. They didn't have farms or supermarkets where they can just purchase their food so they can eat three times a day and in between.

Before they could eat, our ancestors had to hunt for their food. The period between these hunts can be considered as fasting, and it could last for days and even weeks.

It is also noted that animals, even today, will abstain from food if they are sick or not comfortable in their environment. It is a natural human tendency for us to rest and conserve our energy if we feel threatened. Our body has a natural mechanism for fasting.

Ancient Greece

Hippocrates, considered as one of the fathers of western medicine, is said to prescribe fasting alongside regular consumption of apple cider vinegar. The Greek physician is quoted with the following passage:

> *"Everyone has a doctor in him; we just have to help it in its work. The natural healing force within each one of us is the greatest force in getting well. Our food should be our medicine. Our medicine should be our food. But to eat when you are sick, is to feed your sickness."*

Meanwhile, the Greek historian Plutarch also shares the same opinion. He preferred fasting than taking medicine to cure illness. Greek thinkers Aristotle and Plato also believed and practiced fasting. Another advocate of fasting was the Greek mathematician and philosopher Pythagoras.

In other early civilizations, fasting was usually enforced among soldiers before going to war or as part of a ritual. Native North Americans were noted to observe fasting so they can appease their gods and avoid disasters such as drought or famine.

Many of the medical treatments practiced by the ancient Greeks were based on their observations from nature. Similar to most animals, humans don't eat when they are sick. Therefore, fasting was referred to as the internal physician, which is part of our natural instinct to lose our appetite when we are sick. When was the last time you were down with flu? Eating was the last thing in your mind, right?

Fasting was an integral part of ancient healing and has been ingrained into our human psyche. Aside from its healing benefits, the ancient Greeks also believed that fasting can significantly improve a person's cognitive function. When was the last time you ate in an all-you-can-eat restaurant? Did you feel more mentally alert or energetic afterward? Or, rather did you feel a bit dopey or sleepy? Probably the latter, right?

When our stomach is full, our body sends more blood to our digestive system to help in the proper digestion of food and absorption of nutrients. In this case, there will be less blood that goes into our brain, which causes lower mental alertness.

Other great thinkers have also positive sentiments for fasting. Paracelsus, the father of toxicology, said that fasting is the greatest remedy. On the other hand, Benjamin Franklin, one of the founding fathers of America, once said that fasting is the best medicine alongside resting.

Fasting as a Religious Practice

If you are not convinced by philosophers and physicians, maybe great religious figures will do.

Fasting was widely practiced and remains an integral part of the major religions of the world. Mohammad, Buddha, and Jesus Christ all shared the common affinity to the spiritual benefits of fasting.

In the context of spirituality, fasting is usually referred to as purification or cleansing. Different cultures and religions developed fasting independently, and it was not considered as harmful but was beneficial for the body, mind, and spirit.

Buddhism

Practicing self-control is the basis of fasting in Buddhism. Basically, Buddhist monks do not eat any solid food after noon. On the other hand, lay people also abstain from eating solid food after noon (during full moon days) if they are observing the 8 Precepts.

Aside from mastering self-control, fasting is also practiced by Buddhists so they can sacrifice a meal and contribute their food to the poor.

In Buddhist teachings, the struggle against the temptation for food and lust signals the beginning of self-mastery. Also, Buddhists believe that self-control is the first condition of a good life, and so fasting is the first condition of a life that is within your control.

Spiritual sages in different cultures who practiced self-control started with the discipline of regulated fasting. Many of them have succeeded in achieving unbelievable levels of spirituality.

According to one Buddhist legend, a monk was kidnapped and tortured. His feet and hands were cut off upon the orders of a barbaric warlord. However, the monk endured the torture and felt no anger or hatred towards his captors. It is said that the monk has developed his mental power through fasting and self-control.

Christianity

In Christianity, fasting is done by giving up food for a specific duration so they can focus their thought on worshipping God. While fasting, many Christians are praying or reading the bible.

Fasting is also found in the bible for more than 50 times. For example, fasting is depicted in the Old Testament as a way to express grief or to show humility before God. Meanwhile, in the New Testament, Jesus fasted for 40 days in the desert.

In Catholicism, fasting is encouraged during periods of penitence such as Lent and Friday every week. Fasting is also observed by some Catholic communities during the Ember days, and days before major feasts. During the early years, fasting was observed strictly and administered by Church leaders. But over time, this practice became less strict and gradually became voluntary.

In the history of the Catholic Church, the "Black Fast" was observed by strict religious people. This rigid form of fasting was composed of one meal every day that can only be consumed after sunset. Alcohol, dairy, eggs, and meat were forbidden during Black Fast.

During Holy Week, the meals could only be composed of water, herbs, salt, and bread. Catholic fasting gradually weakened beginning in the 13th century with the meal is only allowed during lunch and adding a light snack in the evening.

A morning meal was allowed at the beginning of the 19th century, and in the modern era, Catholics can pray or do charitable work as a substitute for fasting. On the other hand, Eastern Catholics are a lot more rigid in their fasting. They are only consuming one meal every day and they are abstaining from animal products.

In Christian history, it was noted that women seem to have had the strong inclination for religious fasting. In fact, this is called anorexia mirabilis or the miraculous state of not feeling the urge to eat. Those who experienced this can survive an extended period of time without eating and was considered as a sign of chastity and holiness. For example, Julian of Norwich who lived in the 14th century in England used anorexia mirabilis as a way for her to communicate with Christ.

Hinduism

Fasting in Hinduism is part of *Vratas*, which is a religious practice that involves specific obligations. In observing *Vrata*, a Hindu should abstain from eating meat, remain clean, practice forbearance, speak the truth, and perform specific rituals. Once started, a *Vrata* must never be left undone, nor should a Hindu begin another.

Hindus regularly fast twice a month, specifically the sunset before and the sunrise after the moon cycles depicted by Ekadashi. They fast without water and those who worship different Hindu deity fast on different days. For example, those who worship Vishnu fast during Thursdays, while those who worship Shiva fast during Mondays.

An average Hindu can fast for around 36 hours per month.

Islam

Fasting is also an integral part of Islam. Muslims abstain from food and water from sunrise to sunset during Ramadan. Prophet Mohamad also encourages fasting during Mondays and Thursdays of each week.

In the Islamic spiritual context, the purpose of fasting is to develop a deeper sense of righteousness or taqwa. This is done by abstaining from desires and controlling human thoughts.

When fasting, Muslims start with setting a private intention. When the fast is broken, the person should fast another extra day. However, if the fast is broken by sexual intercourse, the person should fast for two months and feed 60 people.

Fasting is believed to bring a Muslim closer to Allah and forges solidarity with your fasting brothers and sisters. It is also seen as a way to understand the struggles of the poor and a way to control human desires. Without spiritual intention, fasting is just considered simply as starvation.

Aside from benefiting the mind and the spirit, fasting is also practiced by Muslims because of its health benefits.

Jainism

Fasting is a common practice in Jainism, which integrates many forms of fasting including abstaining from food to satiation. Jains usually fast by abstaining from food or water, but some are permitted to take boiled water. Jains are also strict vegetarians.

Jains believe fasting is a sure way to keep control of the desires of the body, resolve gathered bad karma, and reinvigorate the soul. While fasting, Jains are expected to read scriptures, meditate, perform charitable acts, and serve the priests.

Judaism

Jewish people fast for at least six days every year. They basically abstain from eating food from sunset to another sunset or 24 hours. Aside from fasting, they also wear leather and prohibited to wash, use perfume or participate in a sexual intercourse, especially during Tisha B'Av and Yom Kippur.

These are only the major religions that include fasting into their spiritual practice and for different reasons. However, they share the same idea that fasting can help not only the body but also the spirit. For some believers, the basic act of fasting can provide them with the power to examine their psyche and stay away from the desires of the human flesh.

It is important to take note that you don't need to practice these religions so you can start intermittent fasting. As long as you follow a regular schedule of fasting (that you will later learn in this book), you can take advantage of the wonderful benefits from this ancient practice.

Therapeutic Fasting

Therapeutic fasting is different from religious fasting. In this approach, fasting is practiced not as part of religion but rather as part to cure or prevent diseases, usually under the supervision of a medical professional. This form of fasting became popular in the US in the 19th century during the onset of the Natural Hygiene Movement.

One American pioneer of this movement was Dr. Herbert Shelton who opened his first health school in San Antonio, TX in the 1920s. By using water fast, Dr. Shelton claimed that he had successfully cured 40,000 patients who suffered from different diseases.

Meanwhile, in the United Kingdom, therapeutic fasting became popular in the 1920s as part of the Nature Cure movement, which also highlighted the importance of positive thinking, breathing fresh air, getting enough sunshine, right diet, and exercise. In Edinburgh, the firth Nature Cure clinic was opened so people can regularly consult medical professionals on how to properly fast and achieve good health. Other fasting clinics were also opened in the UK such as in Hertfordshire and Buckinghamshire.

In both sides of the Atlantic, fasting was used by early therapeutic advocates as a way to treat headaches, allergies, digestive problems, obesity, hypertension, and heart disease. Fasting doctors helped each patient to identify their health condition and follow a specific fasting plan. The fasting clinics had to take a thorough investigation of the patient's' medical history to check if they were suitable and they would be monitored closely.

Therapeutic fasting gradually fell out of favor as scientific medicine became more dominant with the development of prescription drugs. But in Germany, where therapeutic fasting was introduced by Dr. Otto Buchinger, fasting is still popular today and there are still operational fasting clinics around the country. Many German hospitals are still running fasting programs that are even sponsored by health insurance companies.

Fasting in Germany is known as *naturalheilkunde* (natural health practice). It is still popular thanks to its integration in the medical practice. German doctors still refer fasting to their patients if deemed necessary.

Modern Day Fasting

At present, it is normally the physicians and healers with a holistic or spiritual orientation that promote fasting for health and wellness purposes. Natural remedies are still not fully embraced by conventional western medicine.

However, with the gradual acceptance of the body-mind connection, more western doctors are now willing to work with this strong ancient wisdom, trying to not intervene with, but instead to boost the body's own natural mechanism. As Western medicine is looking into this horizon, it will soon rediscover the power of fasting as a remarkable tool for healing.

Scientific studies now support the concept of an invisible energy that is directed through the body, which will naturally attract the body to find balance. For example, Dr. Mehmet Oz, a Turkish-American TV personality believes that doctors should also study the patterns of energy in the body. These unseen energies should be studied further through science so we will understand how we can enhance these for wellness.

Scientists are now looking into new pieces of evidence suggesting that the body is more than biological processes. No advanced medical procedure can treat a body that is not spiritually, emotionally, or physically calibrated for healing. It is only the body that has the natural ability to restore damaged tissues. The natural remedies, on the other hand, can improve the emotional, mental, and spiritual aspects of a person.

Fasting is one great example of this. Even a few hours of fasting can bring wellness not only to the physical mind but also to the human psyche.

Spartans Up!

Discipline is the common factor shared between the Spartan Approach and the religions that encourage fasting. Without following the rigid rules, you may not experience success with this diet regimen. So if you want to get the most out of this, you should know the rules and you should develop the right mindset to follow them.

2

The Story Behind Intermittent Fasting

Our present-day society preaches about the importance of eating three meals daily, with nutritious snacks in between meals. Historically, this is not in harmony with human evolution. The human body is not designed to handle satiation. That is why overeating leads to anomalies such as obesity and the development of diseases.

Many of us believe that skipping meals (especially breakfast) is bad for our health. This is not true, despite the research published correlating breakfast to better health and higher efficiency at work.

However, we should take note that the field of nutritional research is still in its infancy, and many studies that lead to misconceptions that we should not skip meals or deny ourselves with food do not account for important factors.

For example, a massive epidemiological study, which correlates skipping breakfast and weight gain failed to consider variables like highly processed foods during lunch and dinner and high-stress jobs.

In addition, we should also turn to common sense when it comes to addressing the claim that skipping meals affect our metabolism. More often than not, those who are leaner tend to be restrictive of their calorie intake. They know how to control their diet, usually achieving this by skipping meals or fasting.

Obesity is at an all-time high not only in the US but around the globe. We can certainly take advantage from a bit of self-regulation in our food, and when diets are difficult to maintain, probably a strict fasting plan can resolve two major problems – restricting calories without the overwhelming responsibility for a restrictive diet.

This is why there is a boost in the number of research exploring the effects and benefits of intermittent fasting. And for you, this might change your life.

Intermittent Fasting for Weight Loss

In general, fasting will allow the body to eliminate excess fat from its system. It is important to understand that fasting is natural. As already mentioned in the previous chapter, our ancestors didn't have an abundance of food. Hence, our bodies are not biologically evolved to handle satiation. In fact, our bodies are capable of fasting without any serious consequences to health.

Fat is basically a fuel storage that our bodies keep as reserved energy. Even without eating for days, we can still function well.

One fundamental concept of fasting is achieving balance. It is the opposite of eating. When we don't eat, we are basically fasting. Once we eat, our body is absorbing more energy that we can use automatically. But with our less active lifestyle, most of the energy from our food intake is reserved. The main hormone involved in energy storage is insulin.

Whenever we eat, our body is elevating its insulin levels. It also stores fat and sugar in the liver. Through this important hormone, sugar will be converted into glycogen that is then stored in the liver. But there is only a limited space for storage, and once this is achieved, this organ will start converting the added glycogen into fat.

And so, the liver will become the storage house for the newly converted fat. However, most of the fat will be stored in other parts of the body. While this is a complicated process, there is no limit in the amount of glycogen and fat that the body can produce. Hence, there are two main storage processes that happen in our body when we eat. First, is the unlimited storage but hard to access in the form of body fat. Second, is the restricted yet accessible storage in the form of glycogen.

When we fast, our bodies lower the amount of insulin, and the system will start the burning process for fat and sugar. The blood glucose level also decreases, so the body can now use glycogen to burn for more energy.

The human body is designed to easily burn glycogen. This is converted into glucose that provides us with enough energy for the body to burn for at least 24 hours. After this, our bodies will start converting fat into energy again.

Therefore, the human body can exist in two main modes - the insulin low (during fasting) and the insulin high (during feasting). It's either we are burning energy or we are storing it. If there is a balance in the way we eat and feast, then we can avoid too much fat.

Once we start eating the time we wake up, and we don't stop until satiation, we are basically switching our body into insulin high mode. Eventually, we are just building up weight and preventing our body to burn any energy.

Types of Intermittent Fasting

Intermittent fasting has taken off in recent years and so we now have variations of this diet that we can choose depending on your needs and preferences.

The Warrior Diet

The Warrior Fasting is a type of intermittent fasting introduced by Ori Hofmekler - a renowned author and inventor. This diet is based on survival science and advocates a radical diet approach, which challenges common beliefs about fitness, health, and diet.

Basically, the Warrior Diet promotes fasting for 20 hours daily then consuming a hearty meal at the end of the day. Hofmekler claims that consuming a large percentage of calories in the evening is in harmony with how the human body survives and can help a lot in boosting weight loss and muscle development. Take note that this claim is often criticized because of insufficient data from the scientific community.

Other critics of the Warrior Diet say that this diet can be difficult to follow when it comes to working on macronutrients as it can be difficult to maintain our appetite by consuming around 180 grams of protein in one hearty meal.

Be sure to consult your doctor if you want to follow this form of intermittent fasting.

Alternate Day Fasting (ADF)

ADF is a type of intermittent fasting in which you fast and eat in between days. This is mainly a method to lose weight, and so those who want to try this should not increase their calorie intake for those days that they are allowed to eat. With this, you can gradually lower down your weight.

ADF makes sense if you are overweight or sedentary. This is not ideal for those who are hitting the gym as you need the energy to sustain the rigorous training. On the other hand, you may need to increase your intake of protein during minimal calorie periods if you want to minimize muscle loss.

Eat Stop Eat

Eat Stop Eat is a type of intermittent fasting introduced by Brad Pilon. This method is easy to follow but requires longer fasting than other forms.

In this approach, you need to fast for 24 hours at least once or twice a week. You can start fasting on your own pace, but the duration should be 24 hours. While you should not eat food or drink sugary liquids, you can still drink calorie-free beverages like coffee or tea.

The Eat Stop Eat is effective for several reasons. Basically, it is not difficult to follow because you can easily adapt it to your lifestyle. You just don't eat for 24 hours. Meanwhile, similar to most forms of intermittent fasting, the lower caloric intake for extended periods of time contributes a lot for the success of this form. For instance, if you usually eat 2,000 calories daily, this is around 14,000 calories in one week.

If you fast for at least two non-consecutive days, your consumption will be down to 12,000 calories. Without any significant change in your lifestyle, you are on the pace for more than 1 pound of fat every week. Even if you slip up a bit more on your feeding days, you can still wind up with the recommended deficit in your calorie intake. It is not that difficult to see constant weight loss if you integrate some exercise.

Aside from calorie control, this form of intermittent fasting can work really well thanks to the impact of fasting in your general hormonal set-up. In particular, we are talking about growth hormone and insulin.

On insulin, the less often we eat, the less often we increase insulin levels. High levels of insulin in the body can make it extra difficult to lose fat. Therefore, if you are eating less often, you can have minimal issues with your insulin - even if you are consuming the same food and the same caloric intake.

If you think you are not yet ready to fast for as long as 24 hours, then you can begin with a shorter duration like under 16 hours until you can reach the ultimate target of 24 hours.

Leangains

Leangains is another form of intermittent fasting. This was developed by Martin Berkhan mainly for athletes and individuals who need to work on certain body areas.

In this form of intermittent fasting, men are recommended to fast for 16 hours, and then eat during the remaining meals of the day. Meanwhile, women are recommended to fast for 14 hours then eat for the remaining meals of the day. Fasting starts after taking the last meal of the day (usually dinner) and stops with the first meal (usually lunch).

Drinks that are filled with sugar and calories are also to be avoided. Black coffee, sugar alternatives, diet soda, and sugar-free gums are allowed.

Aside from all the benefits that are inherent in other forms of intermittent fasting, the Leangains approach stands out mainly because it provides an advanced way to manage your hormones.

Spartans Up!

The Warrior Diet resonates well with the Spartan habit of fasting. However, this may not be suitable especially for beginners. The next best type of intermittent fasting is Leangains because it is doable and provides an easier approach for fasting compared to the Warrior Diet.

To be sure, consult your doctor first before starting any form of intermittent fasting. Yes, you might be itching to start this plan that can free you from the bondage of being out of shape. But you should remember that a real soldier will never head out into battle without the command from his general.

3

Misunderstandings about Intermittent Fasting

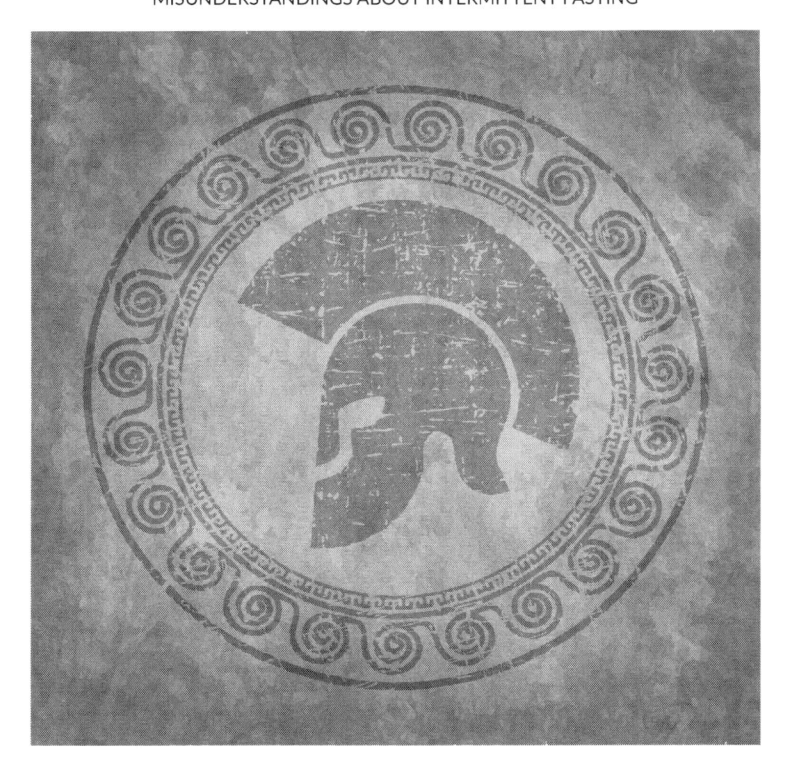

More people who want to lose weight and maintain an ideal body size are reporting positive results with intermittent fasting. As an ancient practice, many modern athletes and bodybuilders are now using this eating lifestyle.

However, there are some people and groups who dismiss intermittent fasting as another health craze or fad. This is despite the substantial historical and scientific evidence that fasting is actually good for the health. In this chapter, we will discuss some common misunderstandings about intermittent fasting.

Losing Weight Is Possible Even Without Calorie Deficit

Many health gurus today are advocating intermittent fasting. They are even promoting it as the fat loss solution of the future. One common claim is that with fasting, there is no need to count calories anymore. Some advocates say that during eating days, you can just eat what you want and you can still lose weight.

This is not true and can even be dangerous for those who want to try intermittent fasting. In order to lose weight, the body needs a negative energy balance. We need to put less energy into our body than we burn to trigger the process of weight loss.

When it comes to getting around the energy balance of our body, there is no magical formula. To successfully lose weight, especially if you want to build muscle mass, you must control your energy consumption. If you want to consider intermittent fasting because someone told you that you can eat as much junk food as you want, then you are misinformed. You still need to restrict your caloric intake during feeding days.

You Need to Fast for Days

Fasting is often associated with absolute starvation, where a person would stay away from eating any solid food for 24 hours or more. This is not the case with intermittent fasting.

In a study conducted by Dr. Krista Varady from the University of California Berkeley, she discovered that lab rats who consumed 25% of their daily calories in one day failed to consume 175% the next day. The rodents started losing weight because they were not completely compensating for the absence of food.

When this method was adapted to humans, the average consumption was only around 115% of their daily caloric allowance during feed days.

If your recommended caloric diet is around 2,000 calories, fasting could be cut down to about 500 calories. You can further decrease this limit if you want to lose more weight. But be sure to check with your doctor first before pushing your limits.

Intermittent Fasting Could Lead to Severe

Health Conditions

Many people who are following a certain diet find it difficult to follow with the restrictions. Low-calorie diets can be hard to follow, and missing for just one day could severely affect the metabolism, which harms the body and affects the effort to lose weight.

Intermittent fasting, according to research conducted by the Brazilian Medical Association, has been shown to be easier to follow compared to other diet systems. This provides a regular negative energy balance in the long run.

The researchers believe that the primary effect of intermittent fasting is how it improves the body's response to insulin, which is the hormone that is crucial in regulating blood sugar. Recent studies reveal that the body is more capable for insulin response while on intermittent fasting.

Individuals who are clinically categorized as obese usually have more difficult time regulating insulin. This is often associated with heart failure and diabetes. Intermittent fasting can help in the prevention of numerous diseases because it helps people to eat less and lose weight. But take note that there is still no hard evidence that by itself intermittent fasting can decrease or increase any form of diseases.

Intermittent Fasting May Cause Muscle Loss

The main reason behind why the body loses muscle mass during an extreme diet is because, after a specific period, our bodies need to use the energy stored in the muscles to sustain our needs. Our body is just responding to the lack of energy supply from calories or carbohydrates so it will start breaking down muscle tissues

This process is known as a catabolic process where the muscle tissues will be consumed by the body. This involves a sub-process known as DNG or De Novo Gluconeogenesis, in which the amino acids in the bloodstream are broken down into glucose. If the body is no longer able to trace these amino acids (caused by long-term fasting) it will turn to muscle tissues.

Muscle loss should not be a concern when it comes to intermittent fasting. If the body needs to sustain muscle tissue, it doesn't require a regular supply of amino acids. There is no need to worry about these complications if the last meal before the onset of fasting was well-balanced and enough.

As such, going into fasting for several hours will not trigger the protein synthesis in the body. Thus, it is important to take note that you will also not gain muscle in this period.

In a research published by the American Journal of Clinical Nutrition, it was discovered that intermittent fasting resulted in zero muscle loss after 56 days. The study participants lose around 5.6 kilograms, which are all from stored fat.

Intermittent Fasting Causes Nutritional Deficiencies

The primary concept of intermittent fasting is in training the body to eat during specific intervals instead of all throughout the day. The absence of food for several hours will not cause any form of nutritional deficiency. The human body is not that weak.

You can still eat again the next day, and in some instances after a few hours. You will be fine if you are maintaining a balanced and healthy diet during your feed days.

If you are still worried, you can consult a dietitian. You can also try taking vitamin supplements to make sure you get enough nutrients. Some people also limit their fasting days to two days a week rather than every other day. Intermittent fasting is not a dangerous practice for cleansing your body. It is about training the body to control our desire for food and avoid overeating.

Intermittent Fasting Could Cause Eating Disorders

You are probably not fit to try intermittent fasting if you think that you can't follow the discipline of proper diet and workout regimen. Intermittent fasting is a regimen used by athletes and bodybuilder. This is not for couch potatoes.

Some people claim that they developed an eating disorder when they tried intermittent fasting. More often than not, those people who are attracted to new diet regimens are more vulnerable to eating disorders.

Usually, those who developed eating disorders are people who overeat during feeding days thinking they can forge themselves with unhealthy food because they will starve themselves the next day.

This is not the purpose of intermittent fasting. You still need to be disciplined and responsible in what you are taking in during feed days. Intermittent fasting may not be the eating habit for you if you are prone to emotional or psychological disorders, especially if you have a record of eating disorders.

It can be easy to avoid these complications if you follow the rules of intermittent fasting. The idea is to maintain a proper negative energy balance for weight loss. Like a Spartan, you need to be disciplined and be conscious of what you eat.

Intermittent Fasting will Make You Weak

In a research conducted by Dr. Varady, she asked several groups of individuals to wear accelerometers to measure their activities. One group are told to follow intermittent fasting, another group is consistent in their daily calorie consumption, while the other group was not restricted in their diet. The research recorded no statistical difference in the everyday activities of the subjects.

During the first week of following intermittent fasting, the group was less motivated to exercise. But after they resumed exercising, they achieved the same level of performance as they did before they go into fasting.

However, the significant discovery of the research is that it is ideal to exercise in the morning during fasting days. The fasting group was able to lose more weight when they exercise in the morning prior to their fasting compared to those who exercise during feed days. Dr. Varady linked this on the impulse to eat a snack after a workout.

Intermittent Fasting Is not Healthy Because

It Promotes Skipping Breakfast

Many of us still believe that breakfast is the most important meal of the day. This is not true and actually the result of commercialism, rhetorical moralization, and sheer advertising.

Our belief that we should start a day with a bowl of cereal or fried bacon and eggs is actually a recent phenomenon. Prior to the 19th century, Americans didn't have that kind of reverence. This was changed by lobbyists for bacon and cereal companies alongside religious fanatics.

According to Abigail Carroll, the author of the book "Three Squares: The Invention of the American Meal", breakfast before the turn of the century was not associated with any type of food. Americans just ate whatever they want in the morning. Usually, these were leftovers from dinner.

By the 19th century, the typical farmer's breakfast (composed of eggs, bacon, and bread) started showing up. Eggs are ever popular breakfast item. At farms, they are readily available as chickens lay eggs early in the morning, and it is very easy to prepare eggs.

Meanwhile, chicken meat was never an item for breakfast as it is very unlikely that people would slaughter chicken first thing in the morning. However, bacon that was previously slaughtered became popular.

By the early 1900s, people started to experience indigestion. At the onset of the Industrial Revolution, people moved from farms to the city where most of their time was spent standing or sitting in one place. Farmer's breakfast was blamed for indigestion, and so there was a demand for a lighter version.

Seventh-Day Adventist (SDA), a newly formed religion at that time, promoted breakfast cereals. The members of the SDA established sanatoriums where they introduced specific health regimens such as vegetarianism and consumption of whole wheat as a way to prevent diseases. This movement resulted in the invention of the first cereal by James Caleb Jackson. Eventually, Kellogg's (a more popular brand) was also invented from a sanatorium opened by SDA.

Both men were religious fanatics. In fact, Kellogg advocated against masturbation as an evil practice that can be prevented by eating bland healthy foods such as corn flakes. And so, how people thought about breakfast was changed because of moral rhetoric to sell the idea of a healthy morning meal.

This moralization was not only around health and religion. It also involved the American reverence for hard work. By the 20th century, people believe that efficiency and productivity at work can be achieved by eating a healthy breakfast.

The early days of the cereal for breakfast triggered the cliche that breakfast is the most important meal. And after the discovery of the vitamins, breakfast cereal brands began fortifying the corn flakes with vitamins and promoted it as the source of nutrients. Through advertisement, the importance of breakfast was solidified into people's minds.

By 1940s, women were also encouraged to enter the workforce to support the war. Mothers needed to prepare something fast and healthy to feed their children in the morning. This need was filled in by morning cereal.

It was the mix of advertising, rhetorical moralization, and fear of developing diseases that helped pushed the perception of breakfast as the most important meal of the day. However, it was the cunning campaign to sell more bacon that really cemented the concept.

Edward Bernays, a Public Relations expert working under the Beech-Nut company strategically used the health fad to help the company sell more bacon. Bernays (who also claimed that he was a nephew of Sigmund Freud) convinced a doctor to agree that a heavy breakfast composed of eggs and bacon was healthier compared to light breakfast. He then sent this statement around 5,000 doctors across the US for signatures.

The petition was published by newspapers as if it was a valid research. This brought eggs and bacon back into fashion and reinforced the idea that breakfast was not only essential but also recommended by doctors.

Should You Skip Breakfast When Fasting?

According to a 2010 study conducted at the Medical University of Warsaw in Poland, those who eat breakfast have the tendency to be healthier and leaner. However, it is also noted that those who eat breakfast in comparison to those who skip breakfast are more likely to eat a balanced diet, consume less alcohol, more physically active, and non-smokers. Hence, there is the possibility that the health benefits of breakfast advocates are mainly caused by healthier lifestyles.

It is good to know that there are available data to figure out what is really happening. In a project called Bath Breakfast, researchers studied 33 volunteers and compared the effects of eating breakfast and skipping the meal for 42 days. The researchers measured daily caloric consumption, body weight, and other metabolic indicators. With this, they were able to look into the volume of food they take, their energy expenditures, and the long-term effect on their weight.

They discovered that skipping breakfast really decreased the number of calories that the volunteers consumed daily. But it also turns out that they failed to lose weight because they were not physically active enough.

Skipping breakfast is not a guarantee that you will lose weight, especially if you skip breakfast and lunch so you can gorge on a big meal at the end of the day. Again, you should be responsible.

Fasting has its benefits. In relation to fast, the 2016 Nobel Prize in Medicine was bestowed to Dr. Yoshinori Ohsumi for his work on autophagy - a process that consumes broken proteins, pathogens, and other cellular materials that interferes in the proper functioning of cells. This process is triggered by fasting.

Just to be clear, intermittent fasting doesn't necessarily mean you should skip breakfast. Timing is crucial and you should be responsible for watching out for your fasting and feeding windows.

At the laboratory, when rats are only provided with food for eight hours daily, the researchers noted significant health benefits such as higher insulin sensitivity, lower cholesterol levels, and lower body fat. It is crucial to take note that these health benefits are evident in the 8-hour feeding window that coincides during the time when the animals are active and awake.

In comparison, if the feeding window was restricted to a time when the rodents are normally sleeping, they experience unstable blood sugar levels, increased weight, and other bad health effects.

This is also true with human subjects.

In a 2013 study published by Tel Aviv University, obese women who consumed beyond their recommended daily intake in the morning had recorded better improvements when it comes to blood lipids and sugar compared to those who consumed breakfast after lunch.

Skipping breakfast is entirely your choice. Even if you choose to eat breakfast, a shorter feeding window can still do wonders. If you want to try intermittent fasting, you may consider eating earlier in the day, instead of trying to gorge on food later in the evening.

Hence, rather than assigning your feeding window between 1 in the afternoon and 9 in the evening, you may change your feeding window between 9 in the morning and 4 in the afternoon. With this, you can still take advantage of the health benefits of intermittent fasting, while eating in a way that is advantageous for your metabolism.

Spartans Up!

Most critics of intermittent fasting are often those who are promoting another diet regimen or those who are simply too lazy to explore this effective lifestyle. We have busted here the myths and misconceptions about intermittent fasting so that you will be armed with the knowledge. You are on the right path, and you should not allow naysayers to discourage you from achieving your goals. Remember, you are a Spartan. Go hard or go home. And home is not an option.

4

Why Intermittent Fasting Works?

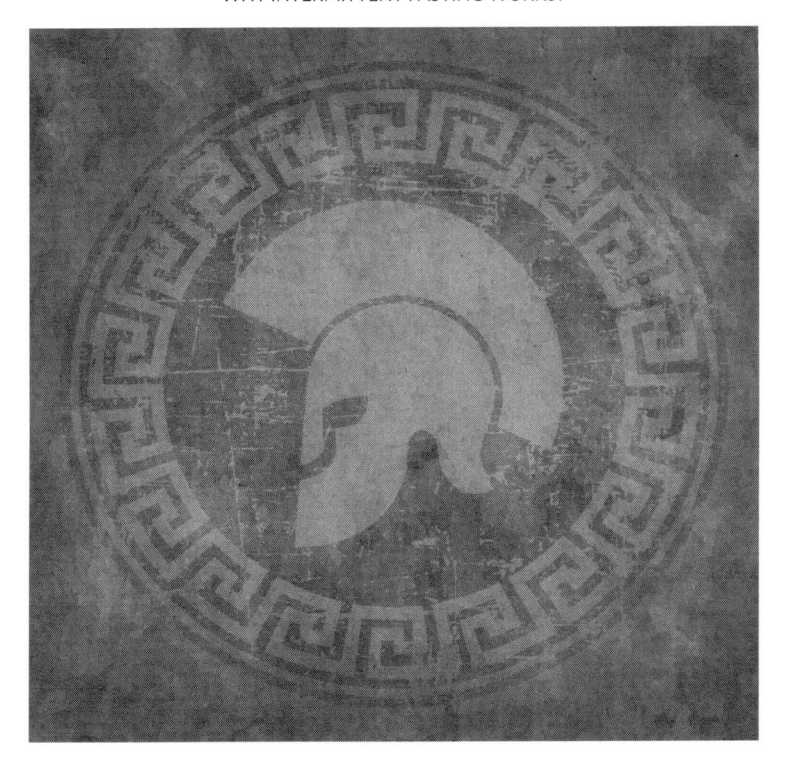

One common reason often cited by supporters of intermittent fasting is that this practice is well-grounded with human evolution. Thousands of years ago, food was not readily available. Our ancestors had to hunt for hours and even days just to find food. If the hunters of the tribe are successful, there will be a feast with meat that is high in calories and protein. But if the hunt failed, the tribe has to skimp on foods that are low in calories such as roots and berries.

This dietary lifestyle has resulted in biochemical and metabolic adaptation through the natural selection process. Through evolution, our species can survive even without the constant availability of food.

The human requirement for carbohydrates, fat, and protein are basically the same with chimpanzees, gorillas, and bonobos. These animals did not have to adapt to intermittent supply of high-calorie food. But there is one important adaptation that impacts the outcome of fasting. This practice can lower our metabolism. Because of the irregular supply of calories, our bodies have learned how to preserve energy.

Studies Supporting Intermittent Fasting

There are different studies that support the health benefits of intermittent fasting. But take note that these studies were performed on lab rats. Human testing has not been carried out. However, the results are still noteworthy.

Based on a study conducted by Mark Mattson at the United States National Institute on Ageing, fasting can help in preserving memory and learning, improve bioindicators of disease, and reduce oxidative stress.

Dr. Mattson performed numerous studies to explore the health benefits of intermittent fasting particularly in the hearts and brains of rats. He is also advocating for a controlled study on human testing that involves various people with various body types.

Dr. Mattson concludes that there are several possible scientific explanations why intermittent fasting is beneficial for human health. One reason that he noted is the hypothesis that during fasting, our cells undergo stress. In the process, the human body is adapting to the stress by enhancing our capacity to cope with the stress and also become stronger in warding off diseases.

While the word "stress" is often seen in bad light, letting our mind and body to undergo mild stress has actual health benefits. For instance, regular exercise places the cardiovascular and muscular system in stress. As long as you allow enough time for recovery, your heart and muscles will become stronger. Likewise, cells can respond in a similar manner. The human cells are designed to adapt the stress brought by fasting.

Dr. Mattson also participated in other research on intermittent fasting and caloric restriction. In one clinical study, obese adults who are suffering from mild asthma consumed only 20% of their caloric intake in between days. The subjects who participated in this control group lost about 8% of their original weight after two months. They also experienced a substantial decrease in body swelling and oxidative stress.

Meanwhile, Dr. Mattson also collaborated with other researchers to study the impact of regular energy restriction and intermittent fasting on fat loss and various biological indicators for particular health diseases such as breast cancer, diabetes, and other cardiovascular diseases. The research team discovered that intermittent fasting and caloric restriction are effective in improving insulin sensitivity, accelerating fat loss, and improving other health conditions.

Dr. Mattson also explored the protective benefits of intermittent fasting to neurons. It turned out that when we fast for at least 10 hours, our bodies tap its fat storage to provide a constant supply of energy. This is done by releasing fatty acids known as ketones into our bloodstream. This process has been shown to safeguard memory and learning functionality and can improve brain health.

But it might also be true that intermittent fasting is beneficial to health as a result of the lower calorie level in the body. Fasting restricts the body from getting the recommended daily allowance. This can create a surplus of calories instead of a deficit. This is part of the findings from the study of slowing progress of diseases like cancer in rodents. The study was conducted by Dr. Freedland from the Duke University Medical Center in North Carolina.

Dr. Freedland and his team highlighted the fact that calorie restriction without malnutrition is one practice that constantly demonstrates long-term survival for lab rats. In this study on the effect of intermittent fasting on the growth of prostate cancer in lab rats, the animals went into caloric restriction for at least 2 days a week.

During the feeding window, the lab rats had the tendency to overeat. At the end of the study, their weight didn't change at all that counteracts any benefit they experience from intermittent fasting. This suggests that the benefits of fasting will be crossed out if you still overeat during non-fasting days.

In order to improve health, the aim is to lose weight by restricting the total amount of calories you take, rather than focusing on when those calories are consumed. He suggests that the body can lose weight if we don't eat two days a week then still restrict diet for the other non-fasting days.

Brown Fat vs White Fat

There are types of fat stored in the body - white fat and brown fat. The latter is mainly used by the body to store extra fuel and the effective release of body lipids as necessary. Too much white fat in the body results to obesity and type 2 diabetes.

Meanwhile, brown fat is used by the body to burn energy and has been explored by many researchers to find a possible solution for the treatment of metabolic conditions such as obesity.

Some studies suggest that under certain conditions, it is possible to convert white fat into brown fat through the process known as browning. This is now widely explored as a way to fight obesity.

In the study, scientists placed lab rats into two groups - a fasting group and a control group. The first group was not provided with food for 24 hours and was then allowed to eat for the next 2 days. The second group was provided with a regular supply of food. This setup continued for 120 days.

Both groups consumed the same level of calories because the rodents in the fasting group were able to catch up during their non-fasting days. At the end of the research, the weight of the lab rats in the fasting group was significantly lower compared to the lab rats in the control group.

The study also reveals that the lab rats in the fasting group experienced more stable glucose metabolism and increased insulin sensitivity. There were also significant differences such as the fact that lab rats that went into fasting had healthier livers and had less lipid buildup.

It was also noted that the lab rats in the fasting group had a lower percentage of white fat as most of the body fat were transformed into brown fat. And when the researchers used the same experiment with obese subjects, they recorded the same health benefits for just 42 days of intermittent fasting.

The researchers are now exploring the physiological and metabolic changes that sustain the benefits experienced by lab rats in the fasting group - especially the browning process. They suspect that the changes in the immune-related gene channels within the fatty cells are causing the changes.

In particular, during the fasting days, the researchers noted a spike in the vascular growth factor, which helps in the formation of blood vessels. It also triggers macrophages to prevent inflammation. The macrophages boost the fat cells to build body heat and burn stored fat.

Intermittent Fasting and Autophagy

The process of autophagy was accidentally discovered when Christian de Duve, a Belgian scientist, was studying insulin in the 1950s. He dubbed the process as autophagy from the Greek words *auto* (self) and *phagy* (eating). This is the process by which the cells are eating some of its own parts to initiate the cleaning process.

Throughout the '70s and the '80s, researchers started looking at the process, but the huge breakthrough was achieved in 1983 when Dr. Yoshinori Ohsumi discovered the specific genes that can regulate autophagy. He discovered that without these genes, it is impossible to regulate autophagy and the cells are not capable of self-repair. In 2016, he was awarded the Nobel Prize for Physiology or Medicine because this discovery became an important pillar for understanding the function of autophagy in cells.

Intermittent fasting may help in improving the process of autophagy, but before that, we should first explore the benefits of autophagy to the human body.

It turns out that the process can be improved if the cell undergoes stress. If in some way the cell is damaged, deprived of energy or lack nutrients, the mechanism to respond to stress will induce autophagy. So when the body is under stress, the cell function actually improves. Autophagy remains functioning only at moderate levels without the added stress.

By activating autophagy, we can reduce the risk of developing health problems related to health. In the process, this will extend our lifespan. This theory is further supported by a study published by the Journal of Clinical Investigation. This study reveals that things that promote longevity also show increased autophagy.

As another research published by the journal Cells, this is partly because the accumulation of different forms of molecular damage is one characteristic of aging. The researchers noted that among the most promising areas in fighting molecular damage is through autophagy.

Cellular Cleanup

Through autophagy, the cell becomes capable of cleaning its own junk. This results in healthier, younger, and cleaner cells.

The human body is comparable to a little universe. Instead of stars, this universe is composed of trillions of cells with their own purpose in how we live and function. These are composed of different parts that are crucial for cellular functions.

For instance, the mitochondria are considered as the powerhouse of the cell because it generates energy. Cells are also composed of proteins that are important for proper cellular function. They serve as messengers to communicate different information across the body, they perform chemical reactions, and they provide structure to tissues.

While they are very small units, every cell works as a unit that produces power and manufactures products that are crucial for proper body function. These cells are doing their job to make us feel, move, think or virtually do everything we do.

Every cell in the body empowers you to read this book, remember a poem, calculate taxes, write a letter, dance, and practically everything else we do every day even while we sleep.

These microscopic units are working every day non-stop, and they are good at their jobs, especially if they are young. With youth, things just keep on humming without any glitch. All systems are functioning well because everything is brand new. The cells are doing their jobs efficiently and so the body is healthy and full of energy.

But this doesn't mean that every cellular system is working perfectly round the clock. They also get damaged over time because of natural aging or accelerated factors such as disease. While we cannot defy the natural law of aging, we can slow it down, seemingly through autophagy and intermittent fasting.

Through the process of self-eating, the cells will break down specific parts by confining them into vacuoles and absorbing them. Through this process, the cells produce wastes such as oxidized particles, damaged proteins, and dead organelles that should be eliminated from the body.

Without proper disposal, these cellular wastes will not leave the body and will start to accumulate becoming toxic to the cells. This accumulation is an important factor in aging. Cellular wastes could get in the way and can impede the cells from doing their job.

This is usually a jargon you might have already learned from other health books, but it is an important fact that once the toxins damage the cellular machinery, it will speed up the aging process. This will cause your hormones to go haywire, your energy to drop, your body to slow, and your skin to look older.

This is why autophagy is crucial. This cellular process serves as a mechanism for garbage disposal. It takes the damaged parts and eliminates them so they will not impede with the normal functions of the body. If this process is efficient, it becomes our natural defense for self-renewal, which can break down damaged structures so that younger ones can be created. This will result to brand new structures that will enable the cells to function properly.

How Intermittent Fasting Triggers High Autophagy

Aside from skin damage, cellular waste is also associated with serious health conditions such as cancer and Parkinson's disease. This decline in autophagy is regarded as an essential consequence of aging. It is not just the breakdown of our cells that becomes alarming. This is also about the decline of our natural ability to fix this issue.

Autophagy can be induced when the body is responding to stress. A natural way to switch on autophagy is to stress your cells. This can be achieved through intermittent fasting.

The main activator of autophagy is nutrient deprivation. Take note that glucagon is the opposite hormone of insulin. If glucagon level is high, insulin level goes down. If insulin level goes high, the glucagon level goes down. When we eat, insulin level will increase and glucagon level will go down. This boost in glucagon will induce autophagy. This suggests that fasting is the best form of boosting autophagy.

Intermittent fasting is more beneficial than just waiting for autophagy to activate. By boosting the process of self-eating, the body can get rid of all the damaged and old cellular parts. Meanwhile, fasting can also stimulate the growth hormone that tells the body to begin producing new parts. Intermittent fasting can hasten the body's mechanism for renovation.

Before you can accommodate new parts, you need to get rid of the old. Think about renovating your garage. If you have the dilapidated cabinets sitting around, you have to detach them and throw them away before you can place new ones. Hence, destruction is just as crucial as creation. If you just try putting the new cabinets without getting rid of the old, your garage will not be as efficient as you plan it to be.

Intermittent fasting has the potential to really reverse the whole process of aging by eliminating cellular parts and replacing them with brand new ones.

Spartans Up!

Spartans were effective soldiers because they were trained in both physical stamina and mental strength. Regardless if they were alone or part of the army, they knew the importance of setting a strategy to tackle down their enemies. In intermittent fasting, it is crucial that you are armed with the right knowledge so you can formulate your winning strategy. You need to pin this down so you know your direction and help you establish your priorities.

5

The Benefits of Intermittent Fasting

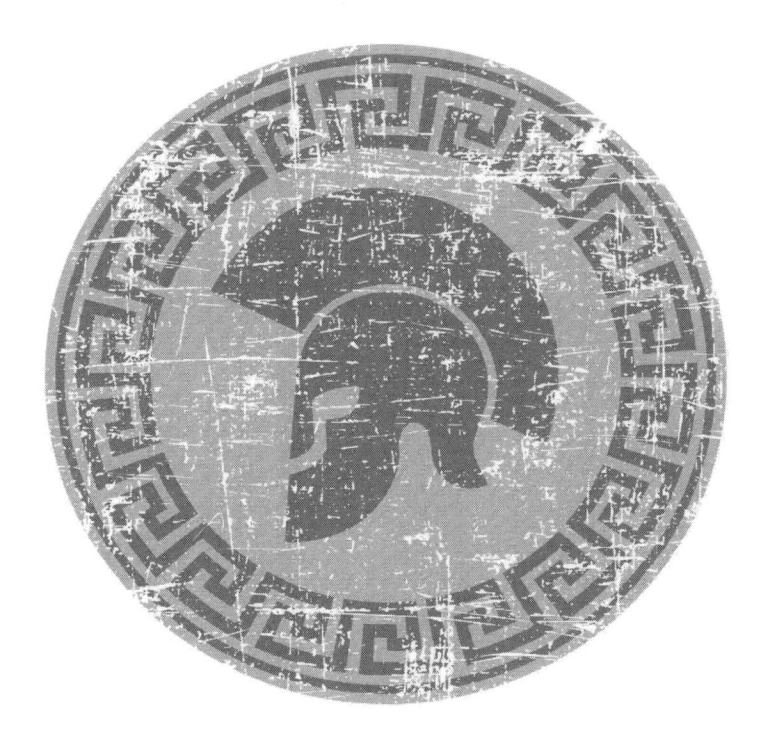

Eating is a basic necessity to live. That is why it can be surprising for some to accept the fact that deprivation from food can be a powerful way to live a healthier life. But as we have discussed in the previous chapters, more evidence are coming to light to support the idea that fasting can have powerful health advantages not only for the body but also for the mind.

As mentioned in Chapter 1, fasting is part of different cultures and religions, and so there are many forms of fasting. Some people can fast for days, while others can only fast for only several hours. Of all these various forms of fasting, intermittent fasting is the one gaining popularity. Celebrities such as Beyonce, Tim Ferriss, and Hugh Jackman have confirmed that they are fasting intermittently. Even executives at Silicon Valley claimed that they have gained more energy and lost weight thanks to intermittent fasting.

In Chapter 2, we have discussed the different forms of intermittent fasting, which makes it quite difficult to classify the practice. The different variations of intermittent fasting are indicators that the bulk of the research showing the health benefits is true for one form but not true for the others.

However, it is still interesting to note that there are promising studies on several types of intermittent fasting, which is a good sign that the benefits of this ancient practice is more than losing weight.

Intermittent Fasting Can Help You Lose Weight

In general, intermittent fasting has gained its popularity nowadays because of its strong promise to help people lose weight. Fasting can drain the body of its glucose storage, which is the primary source of energy from food. In the absence of glucose, the body will switch to ketosis or burning fat for energy.

In a 2014 study published by the journal Cell Metabolism, the researchers discovered that adult lab rats that were limited within a 9 to 12 hour period gained less fat compared to lab rats that were not restricted with their diet. It is also interesting that those lab rats that were allowed access to food during weekends recorded similar results to lab rats that were fasting for seven days. This particular discovery suggests that a short break from fasting doesn't have any effect on the progress.

Another research published by the journal Neurobiology of Disease in 2007 discovered that obese adults who are into alternate-day fasting lost around 5.8 kg after 8 weeks.

Meanwhile, blood samples have revealed that those who fast for at least 12 hours can enter into ketosis, which is a physiological state when the body starts to derive more energy from fat.

The human body gets better at using fat for energy as it enters ketosis more frequently. Hence, some people try to enter into ketosis through keto diets that add a lot of fat into their diets. However, fasting is a considerably more effective approach in improving ketone levels.

You can learn more about intermittent fasting and ketogenic diet in Chapter 9.

Intermittent Fasting Can Improve Blood Pressure

Various studies suggest that intermittent fasting can also help in improving blood pressure.

In a recent study published by the British Journal of Nutrition, the researchers instructed one group of overweight adults to eat normally for 5 days a week and restrict their caloric intake to only 600 calories for 2 days. The other group was told to cut their calories every day.

The two groups were successful in losing weight, but those who only fasted for 2 days recorded faster results. But it is noted that it is not clear if the diet can always help people to accelerate weight loss.

On the other hand, volunteers from the regular diet group had a small increase in their blood pressure, while those who were into intermittent fasting recorded 9 percent drop in systolic blood pressure.

In another study also published recently by the journal Cell Metabolism, researchers deliberately provided the volunteers with enough food that they will not lose weight. They discovered that those who are into intermittent fasting who ate all their calories in one meal improved their sugar levels and blood pressure.

Intermittent Fasting May Help Win the War Against Cancer

A study published by the journal Breast Cancer Research in 2015 reveals that intermittent fasting has an impact on the physical changes that can lead to lower risk for cancer, specifically breast cancer.

The study suggests that energy restriction and weight loss could risk the development of breast cancer cells. The researchers mentioned intermittent energy restriction (IER) as a way to reduce weight compared to equivalent continuous energy restrictions or CER. But it is important to take note that the impact of IER on systemic metabolism and normal breast tissues requires more research.

In another study published by the journal Cancer Cell in 2016, the researchers discovered that the integration of chemotherapy and fasting can slow down the progress of skin cancer and breast cancer.

The integration resulted in the body to produce increased levels of tumor-infiltrating lymphocytes and common lymphoid progenitor cells (CLPs). The CLPs are known as the progenitor of lymphocytes or the white blood cells that can kill cancer cells.

The study also observed that fasting can lead to the production of stem cells and short-term fasting can also increase the sensitivity of cancer cells to chemotherapy.

Intermittent Fasting Can Help Improve Focus

In an evolutionary perspective, being hungry doesn't mean drained or dead. This physiological state is when our brains and bodies need to function at a maximum rate. When we are fasting, we need our brain to function at a maximum capacity, because this is where we need to figure out where and how to find our next meal.

Our ancestors had to be more energetic when they are into the fasting stage because those whose brains and bodies are not functioning well while starving will not be able to survive.

Intermittent fasting can also help in the production of more brain cells, which can affect our brain power. Based on a study from John Hopkins University conducted by Dr. Mark Mattson, fasting has been noted to increase the rate of neurogenesis in the brain. The process of neurogenesis refers to the development and growth of new nerve tissues and new brain cells.

By increasing the rate of neurogenesis, we can increase our focus, enhance our mood, improve our memory, and increase our brain performance. One study published by the Journal of Cerebral Blood Flow & Metabolism reveals that intermittent fasting improved the creation of new brain cells.

Some Forms of Intermittent Fasting May Help with Diabetes

Periodic fasting was the focus of recent studies on the impact of intermittent fasting on diabetes. Researchers from the University of Southern California, led by Valter Longo, started testing if periodic fasting can help diabetic lab rats.

The researchers used mutated lab rats that didn't have leptin, which is a fat hormone that regulates food intake. These lab rats tend to overeat and so they are prone to diabetes and obesity.

The study noted that after several months of periodic fasting, the diabetes was cured by alternating seven unrestricted feed days with four restricted fasting days. The result was promising, but the reason behind it was even more amazing.

Of course, weight loss helped in curing diabetes, but the researchers noted that periodic fasting directly targeted the pancreas. Remember, diabetes is a health condition that is characterized because of excess glucose or sugar in the blood. This is basically a problem with insulin resistance.

In normal conditions, insulin helps cells in the body to absorb glucose from the blood. If the body becomes diabetic, glucose will stay in the blood because cells can no longer absorb it. Partially, this is caused by cells losing their insulin sensitivity. However, this is caused by the inability of the pancreas to stop producing insulin.

The researchers noted that periodic fasting can trigger the pancreas to begin producing insulin again. Fasting provided the pancreas a break, which enabled it to eliminate and reuse many of its cells. Once the lab rats began eating again, new cells that have the capacity of producing insulin were generated.

Hence, the pancreas basically decreased its size during the restricted feed days and regenerated during the unrestricted feed days. The pancreas was nearly good as new with the regular cycle of shrinking, reusing and regenerating.

Of course, we should remember that this research was done on lab rats. There is still no hard evidence that this is also applicable to humans. There is no clear answer yet, but the initial findings from another study conducted also by Dr. Longo seem promising.

In the new phase of the research, 100 volunteers underwent a cycle of 30-day periodic fasting. Each person is provided with 25 days of unrestricted feed days and five days of restricted fasting. At the end of the third cycle, those who began the trial with an increased level of blood sugar noted significant improvements. It is also worthy to take note that none of the volunteers in the trial experienced any adverse effects.

Intermittent Fasting Promotes Longevity

Some forms of intermittent fasting have been linked with considerably improving the human lifespan as well as healthspan. The latter refers to the period that an organism is healthy.

This data has been observed among animals that are in caloric restriction, which limits the number of calories that the animals are allowed to between 20 percent and 30 percent. Take note that there is still no strong data backing up the claim that this can also work for humans.

Meanwhile, a study published by the University of Chicago reveals that intermittent fasting will enable the body to slow down the development of fatal health condition. There is now initial evidence showing that those who regularly fast can experience a healthier and longer life compared to those who are not into fasting or those who are following a conventional calorie restrictive diet.

In an interview, Dr. Mattson again from the National Institute on Aging said that the mild stress that fasting puts on the human body triggers a constant threat. This can increase the body's strong cellular defenses against possible damage in the molecular level.

Intermittent fasting can also trigger the body's mechanism to repair and maintain tissues. The anti-aging properties of intermittent fasting can keep every organ, tissue, and cell in the body to efficiently and effectively function.

Extensive Research Still Required on

Various Types of Intermittent Fasting

Certainly, it seems promising to think that fasting can be a survival mechanism since the dawn of man. The different studies discussed all throughout this book suggest that intermittent fasting triggers the body's healing processes.

However, this doesn't automatically mean that all variations of fasting are the same or that they can provide you with the same health benefits discussed in this Chapter and in this book. The effects will still vary from one person to another, and you must not fail to regularly consult your doctor before you try any abrupt changes in your diet such as intermittent fasting.

You should be cautious in trying intermittent fasting. Of course, different forms of fasting such as eating only during specific hours can provide health benefits. However, extensive research is still needed.

Still, common forms of intermittent fasting are considered now as safe for those people who don't have special health conditions. If intermittent fasting seems appealing to you, and you have already consulted the opinion of your doctor, then this health regime can be worth a shot.

Spartans Up!

Spartans always gave their best shot. They never gave up in the face of adversities because they understood what they were fighting for - freedom from their invaders and glory in the battlefield. Similarly, by understanding the benefits of intermittent fasting, you will be aware of your reward. If you are willing to sacrifice a few meals and follow the strict rules of fasting, you will enjoy living a healthier and longer life.

6

Can You Build Muscle with Intermittent Fasting?

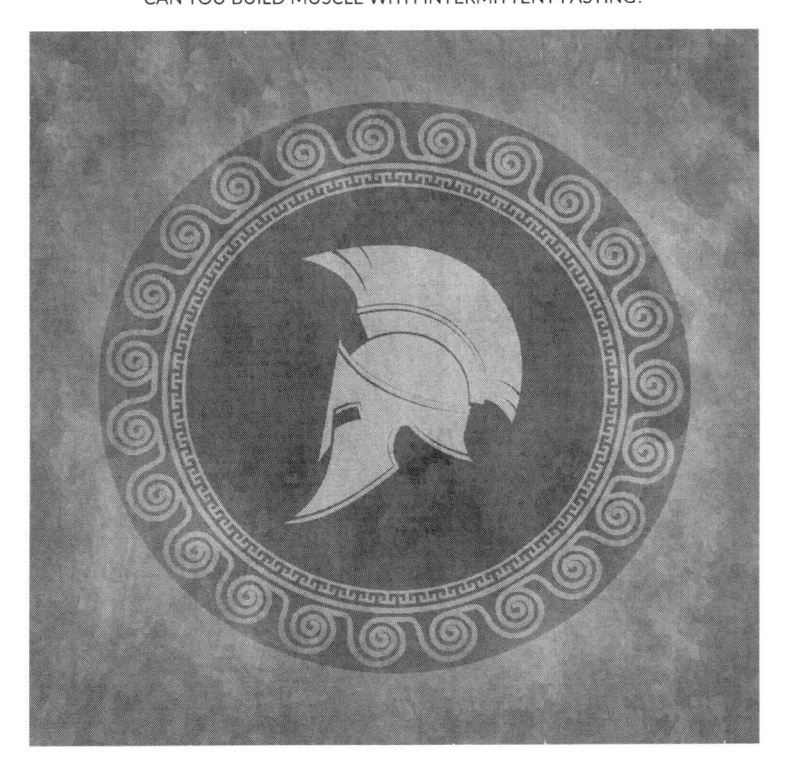

There are not enough studies related to muscle gain during intermittent fasting. This is possibly because weight loss is the common subject of interest in most research concerning this diet regimen.

But there is one study that correlates intermittent fasting to weight training. This study provides vital information about muscle gain. The study involved 18 young adult males who underwent an eight-week training program. The volunteers had not previously performed any form of weight training before the study.

The study volunteers followed either a time-restricted or a normal diet program. For four days, the volunteers were required to take their food within a four-hour period.

At the end of the study, the group on a time-restricted diet had increased their strength and achieved lean body mass. Meanwhile, those who are on a normal diet gained around 2.4 kg of lean mass, alongside increased strength.

This suggests that intermittent fasting is not ideal if you want to gain muscles. This is probably due to the fact that the group who are in a time-restricted diet consumed less protein compared to those who are in a normal diet. However, if we take a closer look into the science behind muscle gain, we can possibly say that muscle gain is still possible while fasting.

The Science Behind Muscle Gain

There are three important factors that should be met in order for a person to build muscle regardless of the training style or diet type:
- The body should have enough resources for recovery
- There should be a positive nitrogen balance so the body can synthesize protein
- There should be enough stress so the body can achieve hypertrophy

The concern whether intermittent fasting can help in muscle gain depends if the body can achieve the three factors above while following a restricted diet.

For the body to have the required resources to repair muscle tissues and achieve maximum recovery, the energy consumption should be higher than energy expenditure. Take note that energy balance has no correlation whether we are consuming 2 meals a day or 12 meals a day.

Consumption of enough protein every day is important if we want to ensure positive nitrogen balance. As long as we are able to consume enough calories during our feed days, then there is no reason why we can limit ourselves from getting enough protein.

So far, progressive overload is the primary approach that we can use to trigger the growth of new muscles. You can do this by increasing the tension placed on the muscle through volume.

There are several ways that we can attain progressive overload, but the main two are adding repetitions without compromising the sets or weight and increasing the weight of the bar without sacrificing the sets and reps. Because it is possible to provide the body with enough energy for rebuilding and recovery, there is no reason that we would have issues when it comes to increasing your performance.

And so, it is safe to say that muscle building through intermittent fasting is possible for anyone who can manage well their calorie consumption.

As you should already know by now, intermittent fasting provides amazing health benefits. If you are still reading this book, I'm sure that you are already hooked into learning more about these health benefits, and you are probably curious if this diet regimen can help you with muscle gain. So let's discuss more intermittent fasting in the context of gaining muscles.

Production of Growth Hormones

Intermittent fasting can trigger the increase in growth hormone production. In a study published by the Journal of Clinical Investigation in 1988, researchers discovered that the increase could be as high as five times.

The evidence is also quite clear that even when growth hormones are injected to increase resting rates, the impact is minimal for muscle gain. So there is still a need for more extensive research to look into how eating patterns such as intermittent fasting can produce physiological changes in muscle mass.

Insulin Sensitivity During Fasting

Remember, the primary role of insulin is to make sure that cells are absorbing the nutrients they need for proper functioning. During satiation, the insulin level is increased, so it decreases the body's ability to break down fatty acids. This makes it more difficult to burn body fat.

Hence, if you are training while on a fasting period, you can burn more fats during the workout. This could mean less fat gain during the bulking phase for those who are in a caloric surplus.

This is an amazing muscle gain benefit theoretically, and also great if you view it from a practical perspective. For most people, training while on a fast could inhibit performance. This could not be an ideal tradeoff if you are hitting the gym for performance. If you want to build more muscle, then you should choose performance over burning fat.

Diet Options

Let's say Mike and Jake are both on a 3,000 kcal diets. Mike is following a conventional approach to eating while Jake is on intermittent fasting. Mike consumes his 3,000 kcal in six meals while Jake reached his target with only 2 meals. In this scenario, it is safe to say that Mike has more options when it comes to selecting foods to include in his diet while achieving his target.

Testosterone Levels

A research published by the Journal of Clinical Endocrinology and Metabolism reveals that the levels of leptin decrease through intermittent fasting. This results in a sudden surge of testosterone. Hence, it is safe to assume that intermittent fasting can boost levels of testosterone in the body.

It is a fact that men who produce testosterone between 300 to 1,000 mg/dl of testosterone are considered to be within the normal level. It is also now a known fact that there is no significant difference in the rate at which the body is building muscles despite being on either higher or lower end of the range.

Moreover, it isn't until the levels of testosterone reach the normal range by 20 to 30% that the muscle growth rate is increased. There is no natural way to achieve this ultimate physiological level yet.

Long-Term Muscle Growth

Many bodybuilders tend to become reckless when it comes to their diet once they have achieved their target for bulking up. This can easily result in a faster fat increase and, ultimately, lower the duration of their bulking phase. It can be difficult to restrict your calories to minimize fat gain while bulking especially if you have a huge appetite. If this is true to you, then intermittent fasting can be an ideal way to prevent overeating when you need to eat to bulk up.

In this case, intermittent fasting may not be ideal to follow if your reference point is the hormonal response. You may choose to try intermittent fasting for a few weeks if you are curious by your body's ability to gain less fat while eating. Try to check how your body will acclimate to the training while still on fast. Check if this regimen is sustainable for you.

Go for intermittent fasting if you can sustain the performance while still fasting. Don't endanger yourself by pushing this regimen if clearly, it is not sustainable in your case.

Calorie Counting

Consumption of extra calories is important if your goal is to build muscle mass. However, for most people, estimating the caloric consumption can result in inconsistency in the regular intake. Failing to track calories each week could add up to your fat gain.

While some advocates of intermittent fasting say that calorie counting is not needed, you should still track down your calories if you want to become leaner and cut down weight. More so, calorie intake from the proper macronutrients is also essential.

Carbohydrates

The human body breaks down carbohydrates into glycogen, which is the main source of energy for strenuous activities such as hitting the gym. Your performance at the gym can be better if your glycogen storage is full. Remember, gym performance is the fastest way to trigger muscular hypertrophy. In muscle building, it is ideal to consume at least 1.5 grams up to 3 grams per pound of your body weight every day.

Fats

Fats are important for bodybuilding as long as your intake is balanced and healthy. For example, a healthy intake of fat is associated with reduced body fat mass, increased hormone levels (anabolic), and faster muscle gain. The recommended daily fat intake for muscle gain is around 0.3 to 0.4 grams per pound of your bodyweight.

Protein

Protein serves as the building blocks of muscles. Hence, it is crucial that you have enough amount of protein intake when your goal is to build muscles. Inadequate amount of protein could lead to a negative nitrogen balance, which means that you end up breaking down more protein than you are taking, and so you can't gain more muscles. The recommended daily protein intake for muscle gain is around 0.8 grams to 1 gram per pound of body weight.

There is no doubt that intermittent fasting can be a viable approach to muscle building. Some advocates say that limiting calories while you are in a bulking stage, especially if you easily gain weight, is certainly a helpful tool to prolong the time you can spend on overfeeding. You can match this up with the recommended muscle training and you can ensure that you will bulk up.

Meanwhile, if you find it difficult to gain enough calories, restricting the time you can eat can do more damage to your health. It is also a reality that most people are not able to perform well while they are in a fasting state.

Just remember that intermittent fasting is a tool that you can use to achieve some health benefits. Like any diet regimen, it has its advantages and disadvantages. If you are curious about it, try it for at least four weeks before saying that it is for you.

If you would rather take your meals less frequently, and you enjoy feasting at the dinner table, then intermittent fasting can be pleasurable. Perhaps this diet is not for you if you prefer smaller and more frequent feeding times.

But take note that regardless if you are regularly eating throughout the day or you are fasting intermittently, if your goal is to gain muscle, you need to take enough calories, consume enough protein, and sustain adding tension to your muscles via progressive overloading.

Spartans Up!

Building muscles is crucial not only for your physique but also for supporting your body's proper function. Both men and women should make sure that they will still hone their muscles while into intermittent fasting. Remember, even Spartan women trained in discus throwing and javelin because they need to be prepared for the tasks of motherhood. In our case, we need our muscles to fulfill our daily obligations. Sure you need to lose weight but you should do this by losing fat and not muscles.

7

What Are the Effects of Intermittent Fasting

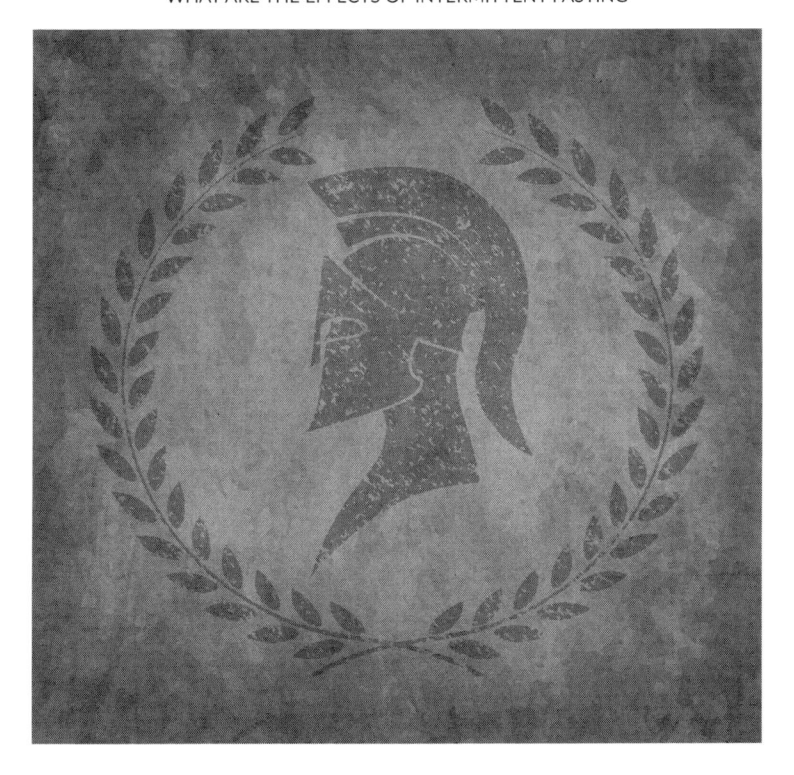

Below are the expected effects of intermittent fasting from your head to your toes.

Smoother and Firmer Skin

Fine lines, spots, and wrinkles are caused by exposure to free radicals that can also damage skin cells. However, fasting can increase the resiliency of cells, which make it easier for them to withstand the damage caused by oxidative stress. This leads to firmer and smoother skin.

Prevent Muscle Loss

While intermittent fasting may not be the ideal diet regimen for bulking up, it has still health benefits for muscle development.

Intermittent fasting can boost fat burning so you can lose less muscle and instead lose more fat compared to other diets. Leaner muscles can help in accelerating your metabolism.

Better Brain Function

Intermittent fasting can boost your mood, promote the growth of new brain cells, and improve cognitive function. Fasting can signal the brain to accelerate the production of protective proteins that can strengthen neural connections.

Healthier Heart

Intermittent fasting can decrease the levels of triglycerides by up to 42% and bad cholesterol by 32%. It also helps in regulating blood pressure. These indicators are important for decreasing your risk for heart disease.

Leaner Liver

Research suggests fasting can fight fatty liver disease. This diet regimen can trigger the production of important proteins that can prevent fat from being stored in the liver and control the absorption of fatty acids.

Powerful Pancreas

After your meals, the pancreas can produce insulin for better absorption of glucose from food and use it for fuel. Intermittent fasting can increase the body's insulin sensitivity, so you need less insulin to process glucose. This will protect you against type 2 diabetes and stabilize blood sugar levels.

Smaller Belly

One exciting benefit of intermittent fasting is the shedding of belly fat. After fasting for at least 12 hours, the body will shift from processing glucose for fuel to burning fat, which includes belly fat. One research discovered that consuming 500 calories every other day is effective for losing weight.

The Side Effects of Intermittent Fasting

It will be chaotic in the beginning. If you are a couch potato, you will not become an athlete with a lean body overnight. The human body requires time to adjust to any form of change. Hence, you are going to experience some side effects if you abruptly change your eating habit. At the onset, these effects may be unbearable, but you can still follow intermittent fasting and enjoy its benefits if you know how to deal with these effects.

Probably you are ready to give this diet regimen a try, but you should be first aware of some side effects that you might experience in the beginning.

Take note that you should check with your doctor first before you begin any new diet plan, especially with intermittent fasting.

Food Cravings

If you learned that you cannot eat chocolate ever again, there is a high chance that all you want to do is to eat chocolate now. When you practice intermittent fasting, you can experience long periods without eating. So there is a chance that all you ever think about is eating. This is when you will experience food cravings.

And because your body is looking for glucose, you will also find that you are more likely to crave for refined carbohydrates and sweets.

To satisfy your cravings, you can indulge in sweets and carbs during your feeding time. You should also find a way to distract yourself from not thinking about food.

Hunger

Your body will expect food at specific times when you are already used to eating at least three times a day. The hormone known as ghrelin is responsible for making us feel hungry.

Hunger typically peaks during meal times and is initially regulated by eating. In the onset of fasting, the level of ghrelin will continue to peak so you will still feel hunger. This will require strong willpower. The first week usually feels the worst, but eventually, you will experience not feeling hungry even though you already reached your feeding window.

The way to combat hunger is to drink a lot of water. This will help respond to the habit of having something to put in your mouth, can help you become more alert, and keep your stomach full.

After 30 minutes of waking up, drink at least 2 glasses of water. If you are still hungry, drink another glass or more. One good thing about intermittent fasting is that you will realize that what you thought was hunger turns out to be boredom or just thirst.

You can also fight hunger by drinking tea or black coffee. Keep busy, get enough sleep, and stay away from rigorous workouts in the first two weeks, because this can increase your hunger.

Another key to preventing hunger is to eat enough during your last meal of the day and get enough fill of protein, fat, and carbohydrates.

Overeating

Some have the tendency to overeat in the onset of their intermittent fasting journey. This usually happens because they experienced cravings a lot so they overeat and ignored the value of controlling their caloric intake. You can avoid overeating if you plan out your meals ahead of time.

You may tend to eat way more than you usually would because you end up eating really fast by the time your fasting ends. You must be mindful of your first meal once you end your fasting. Opt for healthier meals instead of fast food.

Low Energy

You can expect to be a bit sluggish during the first two weeks, mainly because your body is no longer getting the regular source of energy you used to get from eating several times in a day.

To exert the least amount of fuel, try to relax throughout the day. You may want to provide your workouts a break or just perform light exercises such as yoga or walking. It may also help if you get extra sleep.

Headaches

Dull headaches that will come and go will become common as your body is acclimating to intermittent fasting. One factor to consider is dehydration, so make sure that you are drinking enough water both in your feeding and fasting hours.

Headaches may also be caused by stress hormones released during fasting or blood sugar levels decreasing. Eventually, your body will get used to this new diet regimen, but be sure to stay away from stress.

Constipation, Bloating, and Heartburn

When you are not eating, you may experience heartburn while fasting because the stomach produces acid that helps in food digestion. This may range from burping several times a day, mild discomfort, or even pain.

This side effect will eventually go, so just stay hydrated, and avoid spicy and greasy food that can worsen your heartburn. Be sure to consult a doctor if your heartburn doesn't go away.

Constipation is also a side effect of intermittent fasting. This can cause discomfort and bloating. Drinking lots of water can help ease these effects.

Diarrhea

Some practitioners of intermittent fasting also experience diarrhea after their fasting hours. The severity of this condition usually depends on how long the fasting was. Longer fasting may cause mild to severe diarrhea. This is often caused by increased fluid intake.

While you should not limit your water intake (remember, you need to be hydrated during fasting), you can cut down on your coffee consumption. Tea should also be limited to one cup per day.

Feeling Cold

It is fairly common to experience cold toes and fingers while fasting. Don't worry as this comes with a good reason. When you are fasting, blood flow could increase back to your fat storage. This blood flow happens in the adipose tissue, which is important for moving fat to your muscles for burning.

Meanwhile, you can be more sensitive to feeling cold when your blood sugar lowers down. If you are not comfortable with being cold, you can avoid being outside in cold weather for an extended time, wear extra layers of clothing, take a warm bath, or sip hot tea.

Frequent Urinating

Another side effect of intermittent fasting is the increased trips to the bathroom. This mainly happens because you are drinking tons of water to stay hydrated. The bathroom trips could be frequent as once every 30 minutes. There is no workaround for this, as you certainly have to increase your water intake whenever you are fasting. Just make sure that you can easily go to the bathroom when you are in your fasting state.

Irritability

You can be a bit cranky when you need to deal with the other side effects of intermittent fasting such as low energy or cravings. Another cause is when your blood sugar level decreases.

An ideal approach in managing this is by avoiding situations and people that may make you more irritable. Rather, try to focus on doing things that can make you happy.

All these side effects may seem pretty bad, but those who have tried and are successful in intermittent fasting attest to the fact that these usually last for the first three weeks. Easing out into this new diet regimen is the best approach to alleviate its side effects.

Don't be abrupt. Avoid going from eating eight meals a day to eating only one meal. Intermittent fasting can become healthy and natural if you just give it some time.

Although it is also true that not everyone can try intermittent fasting. For instance, children, lactating or pregnant mothers, and people with diabetes should not practice this diet regimen. You should also consult with your doctor before beginning any change in your diet, especially if you are managing chronic health conditions. Moreover, those with history or has a higher risk of developing eating disorders should not try any form of fasting.

There are also instances when the side effects of intermittent fasting must not be ignored. This diet regimen may not be for you if it is leading to the development or unnatural and unhealthy obsession with food, interfering with your capacity to work or live your life, or if you experience a headache due to low blood sugar. You may need to cut your fasting hours and eat a bit earlier as you planned or choose to stop this diet. It is always best to check with your doctor if you have any issues or concerns.

Spartans Up!

Adapting the Spartan Psyche will help you overcome the side effects of intermittent fasting. Many of these side effects are in fact important in the process because every cell in the body needs to experience stress so we can trigger autophagy and start the cleanup process. Once you start intermittent fasting and you experience these side effects, you should understand that these will not last for long. Giving up is not an option. You are a Spartan!

8

An Intermittent Fasting Plan: A Practical Approach

Before starting your plan for intermittent fasting, you should consult your doctor or a health professional if this diet regimen is right for you. Women must be especially careful because there are some mixed arguments whether or not specific fasting protocols are healthy for hormonal balance. Moreover, you need to be extra cautious if you have stomach health issues or you have adrenal fatigue. Again, if you have a history of an eating disorder, you should avoid fasting.

When you begin your fasting journey, you will eventually

experience extended fullness and can simplify the meals you eat. Because there are various ways of fasting, it is ideal to break down each of the various plans into beginners, intermediate, and advanced plans. I have also included the usual daily meals included for each plan.

Remember, a balanced combination of nutrients will provide you with the energy needed to enhance the benefits of intermittent fasting. Just be sure to note any food intolerances you may have, and use the guide for your specific health condition.

The 8-6 Fasting (For Beginners)

In this form of intermittent fasting plan, you can eat between 8 am and 6 pm. Ideal for beginners, this will allow you to still eat the usual meals plus some light snacks in between, but you can fast for 14 hours.

For breakfast, you can try a green smoothie, which is a good way to start the day. A green smoothie is better than a high-sugar smoothie.

Intermediate Plan (For People Who

Have Tried 8-6 Fasting Plan for 2 to 3 Months)

After at least two months of trying the 8-to-6 fasting plan, you can choose to transition to an intermediate level by adding an extra four hours into your fasting. Those who usually skip breakfast may find this plan more helpful. You can just start your day with a cup of black coffee or herbal tea.

In this intermediate intermittent fasting plan, your feeding hours are between 12 pm and 6 pm. This will provide you with a full 18 hours of fasting within the 24-hour period.

Take note that you should stay hydrated despite skipping breakfast. So be sure that you drink sufficient amount of water. You may also drink herbal tea but limit it only to 3 cups per day.

Tea contains a compound known as catechins that help in regulating the hunger hormone known as ghrelin. So by drinking tea, you can make it until lunch without experiencing too much food cravings.

Because you have extended your fasting period with the added four hours, you have to ensure that your first meal (lunch) contains enough healthy fats. For your afternoon snack, you can munch on nuts and seeds. Try to soak the nuts beforehand so you can neutralize the enzymes such as phytates that can result in problems with your digestion. You may eat dinner around 5:30 pm, and then a dinner that is rich in protein is ideal.

The 5-2 Plan (Intermediate Fasting)

For this intermediate intermittent fasting plan, you can eat normally for five days of the week, but you will not eat anything for two non-succeeding days. For instance, you may choose to fast on Sunday and Wednesday but eat normally on the other days.

The quality of food on your feeding days should be like the rest of the intermittent fasting plans. There should be vegetables, fruits, healthy fat, and protein sources. Take note that this plan is not recommended for those who have never tried intermittent fasting. You should always check with your doctor or a health professional before you begin any diet regimen, especially if you have pre-existing medical conditions.

Modified 5-2 Plan (Intermediate Fasting)

This is a modified version of the 5-2 plan, wherein you can choose to eat normally for five days of the week (you have the freedom to choose which days you want to fast). For two days, limit your caloric intake to no more than 700 calories for each day.

Restricting your calories will enable you to unlock wonderful benefits of intermittent fasting. During your feeding days, you need to ensure that you are consuming fruits, vegetables, healthy meat, and fats. You also have the flexibility to structure your meals based on your preference.

During your fasting days, you may choose to have smaller portion of meals or snacks. You can also eat moderate-size meals then fast in the morning or after dinner. Remember, you need to be cautious with the quality of the food you eat. There are helpful apps you can download on your phone to help you record your food and monitor your calories so you will not go beyond your 700 calorie limit.

Alternate Day Plan (Advanced Fasting)

While this plan is considered as an advanced form of intermittent fasting, it is very easy to follow. You just need to fast every other day. This plan can provide you with wonderful results, but this is often reserved for those who have experienced fasting for quite a while.

During fasting days, you can take water, black coffee, or herbal tea. On the other hand, your meals during feeding days should be composed of vegetables, fruits, healthy fats, and a good source of protein.

Hopefully, you now have enough information so you can easily schedule your meals when you want to start intermittent fasting. And though this may seem difficult at first, when you get into this diet regimen, it will become natural to you.

Recommended Foods for Intermittent Fasting

Below is a quick guide on the recommended food items that you should include in your meal plan if you want to try intermittent fasting:

Recommended Daily Servings

Vegetables: 6 to 11 servings
   Healthy fats: 5 to 9 servings
   Animal protein: 4 to 6 servings
   Fruit: 1 to 2 servings

Daily Calorie Allocation

Carbohydrates: 5% to 30%
   Proteins: 10% to 30%
   Fats: 50% to 80%

Or

Fruit: 4%
   Vegetables: 28%
   Animal Protein: 18%
   Healthy Fats: 50%

Vegetables

High

Avocado
   Olives
   Bok Choy
   Collards
   Kale
   Broccoli
   Cauliflower
   Celery
   Dark Lettuces
   Radish
   Green Beans
   Zucchini
   Cilantro
   Parsley
   Brussels Sprouts
   Spinach
   Asparagus
   Cabbages
   Carrots
   Cucumber
   Summer Squashes
   Artichokes

Average

Eggplant
  Tomatoes
  Onion
  Peppers
  Garlic

Low

Beets
  Peas
  Sweet Potatoes
  Yams
  Corn on the cob
  Plantains
  Winter Squashes

Avoid

Canned Vegetables
  Mushrooms
  Potatoes

Protein

High

Grass-fed lamb
   Grass-fed beef
   Protein powders (beef plasma /serum, hydrolyzed collagen)
   Pastured eggs
   Whey protein concentrate
   Trout
   Summer Flounder
   Sardines
   Haddock
   Tilapia
   Sockeye Salmon
   Patrale Sole
   Anchovies

Average

Pastured pork
   Pastured turkey
   Pastured goose
   Pastured chicken
   Whey protein isolate

Low

Factory farmed meat
  Factory farmed eggs
  High mercury fish
  Farmed seafood

Avoid

Soy protein
  Beans
  Wheat protein
  Cooked dairy
  Cheese

Fats

High

Grass-fed butter
  Pastured egg yolks
  Fish oils
  Extra virgin olive oil
  Cocoa butter

Grass-fed ghee
Grass-fed meat fat
Coconut oil
Non-GMO soy lecithin

Average

Palm oil
   Grain-fed ghee
   Grain-fed butter
   Pastured bacon fat
   Unheated walnut oil
   Unheated hazelnut oil
   Unheated almond oil

Low

Duck fat
   Canola oil
   Cottonseed oil
   Peanut oil
   Chicken fat
   Sunflower oil
   Goose fat
   Corn oil
   Soy and vegetable oil

Safflower oil

Avoid

Margarine
    Commercial lard
    GMO grain oil
    Other artificial trans fats

Fruits

High

Blackberry
    Grapefruit
    Lime
    Raspberry
    Cranberry
    Lemon
    Passion fruit
    Strawberry

Average

Apple
   Blueberry
   Cherry
   Nectarine
   Papaya
   Pear
   Plum
   Apricot
   Cantaloupe
   Kiwi
   Orange
   Peach
   Pineapple

Low

Banana
   Grapes
   Fig
   Mango
   Persimmon
   Tangerine
   Dried fruits
   Dates
   Guava
   Lychee
   Melon

Pomegranate
Raisins

Avoid

Canned fruit

Grains

High

None

Average

Brown rice
  Wild rice
  Organic quinoa
  Black rice
  White rice
  Oats

Low

Organic wheat
   Organic corn

Avoid

GMO grain
   Any non-organic whole or refined grains except white rice

Nuts and Legumes

High

Raw coconut
   Brazil nuts
   Hazelnuts
   Pecans
   Pistachios
   Almonds
   Cashews
   Macadamia nuts
   Pine nuts
   Walnuts

Average

Sprouted legumes
- Raw chestnuts
- Green beans

Low

Garbanzo beans
- Peanuts
- Lentils
- Peas
- Dried beans

Avoid

Non-fermented soy
- Soy nuts
- Roasted nuts
- Corn nuts
- Roasted legumes

Dairy

High

Organic grass-fed butter
  Non-organic grass-fed butter
  Organic grass-fed ghee
  Clarified butter
  Non-organic grass-fed ghee
  Grass-fed full-fat raw organic yogurt (non-pasteur and only if you have the tolerance)
  Grass-fed full-fat raw organic milk (non-pasteur and only if you have the tolerance)

Average

Grain-fed non-organic raw milk
  Organic pasteurized milk
  Any cheese
  Grain-fed butter or ghee
  Non-organic pasteurized milk

Low

Blue cheese
   Lowfat milk products
   Skim milk

Avoid

rBGH dairy
   Factory dairy
   Condensed milk
   Ice cream
   Powdered milk

Sugars and Sweeteners

High

Xylitol
   Maltitol
   Dextrose
   Stevia

Average

Raw honey
　Maple syrup
　Brown sugar
　Sorbitol
　Coconut sugar

Low

White sugar
　Cooked honey

Avoid

Nutrasweet (aspartame)
　Splenda (Sucralose)
　Agave syrup
　Fruit juice concentrate
　Aceslsulfame
　High fructose corn syrup

Spices and Seasonings

High

Apple cider vinegar
  Ginger
  Parsley
  Turmeric
  Lavender
  Cinnamon
  Cloves
  Sea salt
  Cilantro
  Oregano
  Rosemary
  Thyme

Average

Organically prepared mustard (no additives)
  Onion
  Black pepper
  Garlic

Low

Fermented soy
  Miso
  Table salt
  Tamari
  Nutmeg

Avoid

Commercial salad dressings
    Spice extracts
    MSG
    Yeast

Cooking Style

High

Raw / Uncooked
    Steamed al dente
    Lightly heated
    Medium baked

Average

Lightly grilled
    Poached
    Boiled

Low

Barbequed
  Broiled

Avoid

Burnt
  Charred
  Microwaved
  Blackened
  Deep fried

Count Your Macronutrients

Calories and macronutrients are just like exercise and diet. It is impossible to achieve your health goals through intermittent fasting if you are not aware of how you can integrate these two with each other.

Take note that calories are made of macronutrients, which makes them important. The three types of macronutrients are protein, carbohydrates, and fat. Basically, these macronutrients contain the following calorie levels:

1 g of fat = 9 cal
  1 g of carbs = 4 cal

1 g of protein = 4 cal

Counting your calories is crucial to keep track of your macronutrients. This is crucial if your goal for intermittent fasting is weight loss. However, there are specific factors suggesting that counting your macros should be a higher priority than counting calories:

- Consuming the recommended amount of fat can boost hormone levels in the body, which aids in better absorption of nutrients from food.
- Consuming the recommended amount of carbs can aid the body to recover from a workout and prevent muscle loss. This is crucial for people who are into intermittent fasting.
- Consuming the recommended amount of protein can aid the body to control hunger, improve muscle development and recover from a workout.

Therefore it is important that you count your macros and take the recommended amount of protein, carbs, and fat.

But how can you exactly count your macros? You must begin with your protein. If you want to sustain your weight, then you should take 1 gram of protein for every pound of your body weight. If you want to lose weight, then you should consume around 1 to 1.2 grams of protein for each pound of your body weight.

After protein, you should work on your fat intake. If you want to reduce fat, then the ideal intake is 0.2 g of fat for every pound of body weight. To sustain your weight, you can increase fat intake to at least 0.3 g for each pound of body weight every day.

Carbohydrates should be your least priority. This macro will just compose the rest of your caloric requirement for the day that is between 30% and 50% of your total daily calories.

Spartans Up!

You can increase your chance for success if you have a plan. Spartans never head into a battle without a sound plan to win. Before you start intermittent fasting, you should choose down the most suitable plan according to your preferences and needs. Be sure to include the recommended food items so you can further increase the benefits you can enjoy with intermittent fasting.

9

What About Keto and Intermittent Fasting Combined?

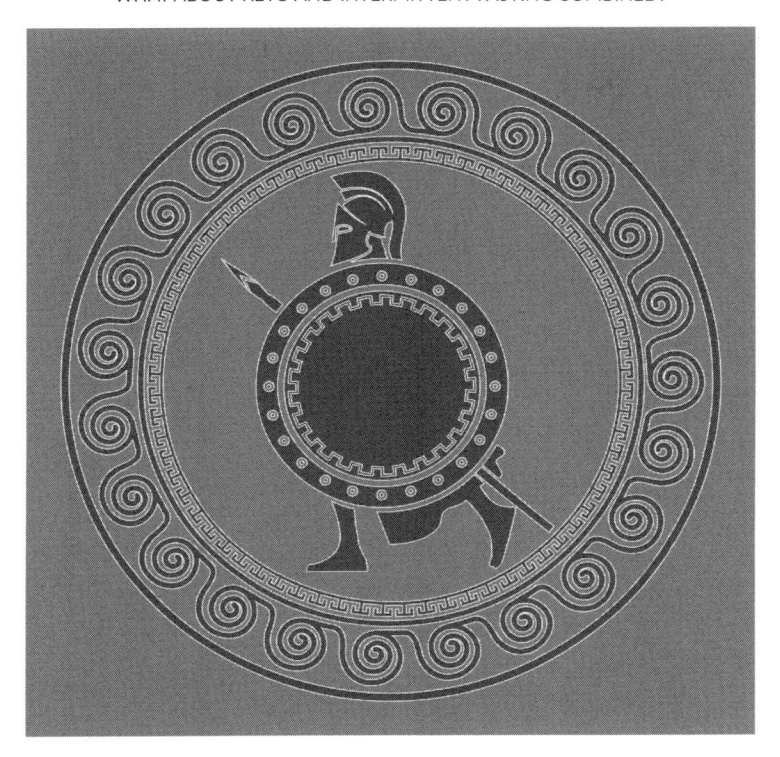

The ketogenic diet is now a popular regimen, which mainly involves specific meal plans and habits to help the body generate ketones in the liver as a source of fuel. Aside from ketogenic diet, this is also known as low carb high-fat diet (LCHF) or simply low carb diet.

If your diet is composed of too many carbohydrates, your body tends to initiate the production of glucose and insulin.

Glucose is known as simple sugar, which the body can easily

convert into energy. Hence, the body will choose to break down glucose first and tap this as the first source of energy. On the other hand, insulin is produced by the body to process the glucose in the bloodstream.

Because the glucose is being used as a main source of energy, the fat storage will be reserved. Usually, in a high-carb diet, the body will use glucose as the primary form of fuel. By decreasing the intake of carbohydrates, the body will switch in a state called ketosis.

The human body prefers ketosis as a primary source of fuel. When there is a limit on its consumption, the body will react similarly to a fasting state. This will induce new energy channels to provide power to every cell in the body. One form of energy channel is known as ketogenesis, and the outcome of this channel is a secondary source of fuel called ketones.

The ketones can be used by the cells in the body except for red blood cells and liver cells. Ketones and sugar affect the body in various ways.

For instance, if the body is mainly burning sugar for fuel, the process will increase oxygen reactivity. This state can cause damage to the cells and even cellular death when they accumulate. That is why high consumption of sugar can affect proper brain functioning and may cause brain plaque.

Meanwhile, the ketones are more efficient to use as an energy source and have been shown to protect the health of neuron cells. This is because using ketones as fuel can improve the production and function of mitochondria and in the process decreases the production of reactive oxygen in the body.

Restricting carbohydrates can also help healthy cells that are struggling to survive. Autophagy will be activated if the body has limited access to carbohydrates. This process triggers numerous factors that can improve the resilience and health of cells, induce processes that stops inflammation and gets rid of toxins from the cells.

Clinical studies reveal that the combination of ketogenesis and autophagy is crucial in helping people with cancer, Alzheimer's disease, migraines, and epilepsy.

The biggest stimulator of insulin will also be taken out of the diet when we restrict carbohydrates. This can reduce inflammation, increase fat burning, and decrease insulin levels. The integration of these three can address the main drivers of several chronic diseases such as fat accumulation, inflammation, and insulin resistance.

Ketosis

The process of ketosis is a natural mechanism of the human body to help us survive if there is insufficient food supply. In this state, the body is producing ketones that are produced from the breakdown of fat deposits in the liver.

The ultimate goal of the ketogenic diet is to induce the body into this metabolic process. This is done through low carb diet to starve the body from glucose.

The human body is highly adaptive, because of its survival mechanism. If we overload it with fats and decrease carbs, the body will start to tap the ketones in the liver as the main source of energy. High levels of ketones in the body provide a lot of health benefits.

There are studies suggesting the benefits of the ketogenic diet over a diet composed of low fat. Weight loss is the primary advantage based on a meta-analysis of low-carb diets published by the New England Journal of Medicine.

Benefits of Ketosis

There are different benefits when the body regularly induces ketosis. This includes increased energy levels, weight loss, and therapeutic medical applications. High-fat, low-carb diet can help almost everyone. Just be sure to seek first the opinion of your doctor or a health professional before drastically changing your diet.

Weight Loss

Similar to intermittent fasting, a body on ketosis will enable it to tap fat as a source of energy. Hence, a ketogenic diet can also induce weight loss. While on ketosis, the insulin level will significantly be decreased that allows the body to burn fat for energy.

Mental Clarity

The ketogenic diet, similar to intermittent fasting, can also help the mind achieve focus. Many people are using ketogenic diet to boost their mental performance. The brain can take advantage of ketones as a great source of fuel. Huge spikes in blood sugar can be avoided when you lower down your consumption of carbohydrates. This can lead to improved concentration and focus. Meanwhile, Omega-3 and Omega-6 fatty acids are also proven to have significant benefits to the function of the brain.

Blood Sugar Control

Because of the type of foods in the ketogenic diet, this regimen can also naturally decrease blood sugar levels just like intermittent fasting. There are also studies that suggest keto-based diet is even a better approach in managing and preventing diabetes in comparison to diets that are based on the low-calorie count. The ketogenic diet is often recommended for those who have pre-diabetes or those who are diagnosed with Type 2 diabetes.

Blood Pressure and Cholesterol

Undergoing regular ketosis can help the body to improve cholesterol levels and triglyceride levels that are usually linked to buildup in the arteries. Ketogenic diet shows a significant decrease in LDL and increases in HDL particle concentration compared to low-fat diets.

Another study reveals low-carb diets can help in managing hypertension over other forms of diet. Hypertension is also normally associated with obesity, which is an added perk because ketogenic diet can result in weight loss.

More Energy

Those who are on ketogenic diet usually report more energy during the day. This is normally due to the fact that this regimen may provide the body with a better and more reliable source of energy. Fats are better efficient source of energy compared to glucose. Furthermore, fat is usually more satisfying and can result in satiation.

Resistance to Insulin

If left unmanaged, high resistance to insulin can result in Type 2 diabetes. Studies reveal that ketogenic diet can help individuals manage their insulin levels to recommended ranges. Athletes can also benefit from insulin optimization on ketosis by eating foods that are rich in omega-3 fatty acids.

Treatment of Epilepsy

Since the early 1900s, low-carb and high-fat diet has been used for the management and treatment of epilepsy. This is still a popular approach for therapies for kids who have uncontrolled epilepsy. Among the primary advantages of ketogenic diet for people with epilepsy is that it allows lower dependence on medications while still providing great control.

Ketogenic Diet and Intermittent Fasting

At this point, you are probably wondering if it is fine to combine ketogenic diet with intermittent fasting.

Well, the answer is yes! These two diet regimens can complement each other well. You can boost the benefits of intermittent fasting by taking ketogenic meals while you are in the feeding window.

Ketosis is the common link between intermittent fasting and the ketogenic diet. Intermittent fasting can drive down the levels of blood sugar in the body. This can trigger or boost ketosis.

While intermittent fasting is not a requirement for the ketogenic diet, it is also not impossible to combine. This is especially true because you are not limiting calories during your feeding window.

But be sure to talk to your doctor if you are diabetic and using insulin and you are on ketogenic diet because you need to manage epilepsy. These conditions require further medical examination to ascertain if it is safe for you to practice intermittent fasting.

Also, make certain that you are taking note of the keto ratios: carbohydrates (5% to 10%), protein: 15% to 30%, and fat (60% to 75%). After this, ensure that your diet is composed of nutritious meals. Avoid highly-processed food items. Most people think that ketogenic diet is composed of meals such as cheese and bacon. However, these foods are quite low in specific nutrients that are crucial for achieving ketosis.

Adding ketogenic diet into intermittent fasting can boost weight loss and fat burn. But take note that the most sustainable and healthiest diet is one that you can really stick to, and ketogenic diet while on intermittent fasting can be difficult to sustain over time.

Spartans Up!

One notable trait of Spartans is their sense of brotherhood. From the age of 7, Spartan boys were trained together, and so they grew up like brothers. They faced the same hardships and they were honed with the same mindset. They were effective as soldiers because they were not only looking for their own interests, but they were also trained to look out for each other.

To win a war, you need allies. To win the war against poor health and obesity, you need allies. Ketosis is an ally of intermittent fasting that you can depend on to further increase your chance for success.

10

Intermittent Fasting and Supplements

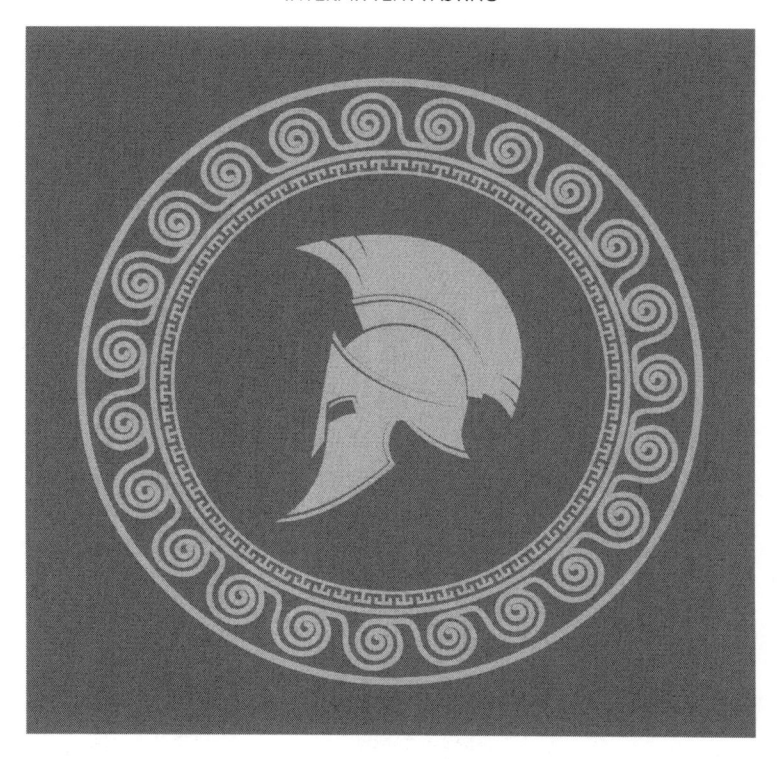

Not all supplements can provide the health benefits you need. Taking the wrong supplements, especially while you are on intermittent fasting, may bring harm. The right types of health supplements can significantly boost the effects of intermittent fasting.

In this Chapter, we will briefly discuss the problems with taking generic supplements, how to choose the right health supplements for those who are into intermittent fasting, and a comprehensive list of health supplements that you should take.

The Problem with Multivitamins

Multivitamins are very popular. Millions of people around the world are taking multivitamins, so people think that they are indispensable for fighting disease and malnutrition. This is, in fact, a misconception. In reality, not everyone can benefit from multivitamins and instead choose targeted supplements.

Nutritional Imbalance

Many multivitamins contain too much of specific nutrients such as Vitamin A or C, and not enough of the other essential nutrients such as magnesium. So there is a tendency to overdose on few nutrients and not taking enough of the others.

Some manufacturers still include a long list of multivitamins on their labels, but the truth is, some of these vitamins are in very small amounts. Many consumers ignore the insubstantial amounts of important nutrients. How can you fit a range of nutrients in only one pill? Also, we need to consider the nutritional needs of each person. A bodybuilder will require a different set of nutrients compared to a lactating mom.

Low Quality of Multivitamins

Each type of nutrient behaves differently inside the body. While folate is an important B vitamin, folic acid – the form found in generic multivitamins, may increase the risk of colon cancer according to a study published by the University of Chile.

This could be the reason why some researches such as a 2009 study published by the University of East Finland suggest a connection between multivitamins and increase in mortality, while another research commissioned by the American Medical Association in 2009 reveals no benefit in taking multivitamins.

Furthermore, many multivitamins are manufactured with additives and fillers, which make it difficult for the body to absorb nutrients. Therefore, a minimal amount of important nutrients may reach your cells.

We are actually getting what we pay for with multivitamins. You may convince yourself and choose the generic multivitamins in the store, or you may add a bit and actually choose targeted supplements to help improve your health.

Supplements and Fasting

Eating whole and natural foods are still the best source to get the important nutrients that our body needs. Remember, whole foods may behave differently from their individual components. For example, the nutrients from a piece of broccoli are more accessible compared to consuming the equal amount of nutrients from a powder or a pill.

The antioxidants sourced from natural foods are beneficial, but consuming mega doses of some synthetic antioxidants may come with risks such as the growth of tumor based on a 1993 toxicology research from the University of Hamburg.

Food synergy enables the nutrients in food to work together. Hence, food is more powerful compared to its components. This is why it is crucial to begin with a diet that is rich in nutrients, then add supplements that are based on your goals and needs.

It is important to take note that just because something is natural doesn't mean it is helpful. There is a tendency for some, especially the health buffs, to abuse even food based vitamins and herbal supplements.

These supplements are still vulnerable from contaminants and heavy metals from manufacturing. Be sure to check the sourcing and quality testing of your supplements. It is ideal to check with a licensed professional who can recommend safe brands of supplements.

Important Nutrients You Should Take

The following is a list of essential supplements that you should take especially if you are into intermittent fasting. For every nutrient, you should take note of the right dosage, the proper form to take, and the ideal time.

Vitamin A

Vitamin A is crucial as a supplement especially if you don't like to eat organ meats such as heart, kidney, and liver. This vitamin is an essential cofactor for different metabolic processes in the body.

The Recommended Dietary Allowance (RDA) for men is 900 µg and 700 µg for women. However, a quarter of Americans consume less than this RDA.

Plant-based diets are poor in Vitamin A because plants don't produce the nutrients needed for the formation of this nutrient. Instead, they have beta-carotene. This is poorly processed into Vitamin A that is why some people develop a deficiency in this nutrient despite taking far more vegetables that they should. Because of this, Vitamin A supplements are crucial for vegetarians and vegans.

The ideal dose is 3000 to 10000 IU per day in the form of retinol. Take the supplement with meals.

Vitamin C

Vitamin C is one of the most effective and safest health supplements you can take. This vitamin is important for the formation of collagen and connective tissues. It can help in eliminating free radicals and improve functions of the immune system.

According to a 2005 study conducted by the Center for the Improvement of Human Functioning in Wichita, KS, the safe dosage for Vitamin C is up to 120 grams daily.

It can be difficult to source Vitamin C from food. That is why around 30% of Americans have Vitamin C deficiency.

Most fruits and vegetables are rich in Vitamin C, but overcooking and long storage may deplete the nutritional content. A daily supplement with at least 500 mg per day is recommended. You can increase this intake (after consulting your doctor) if you are healing from injury or you are experiencing chronic infections.

The usual forms of Vitamin C are in time release capsules or ascorbic acid crystals. It is best to take the supplements in the morning and evening. Avoid taking this after a workout as isolated antioxidants can affect the insulin sensitivity you acquired after gym.

Vitamin D

Vitamin D is another important nutrient, which acts on more than 1,000 various genes and serves as a substrate for hormones such as estrogen, human growth hormone, and testosterone. It helps in the formation of the bones, boost cell metabolism, moderates immune function and prevent inflammation.

This vitamin is a crucial nutrient, in fact, without it, we will be dead. The human body can make its own Vitamin D with enough exposure to sunlight. But for those who are living in areas where there is not enough sunlight, it is recommended to get a Vitamin D supplement. It is also difficult to get overdose from it if you are getting enough Vitamin A.

The recommended dosage is 1,000 IU per 25 lbs of body weight. The usual form is D3 with Vitamin K. There are supplements that provide the three essential nutrients (Vitamins A, D, and K) in one pill. The ideal time to take Vitamin D supplement is in the morning.

Vitamin K2

There is a high chance that you are deficient in Vitamin K2 unless you have been eating only raw milk and grass-fed meat all your life. This vitamin is a fat-soluble nutrient that is crucial for the metabolism of the cells.

The extra amount of calcium in the body can be deposited in arteries, which cause decreased vascular function and calcification. That is why this supplement can lower your risk for bone loss and developing cardiovascular disease.

Vitamin K1 is the form of Vitamin K that is usually found in green and leafy vegetables. Meanwhile, Vitamin K2 is the form that is found in grass-fed meat. Animals such as sheep and cows can efficiently convert Vitamin K1 into K2 thanks to their well-designed digestive system. The human stomach is not as efficient in converting K1 to K2. Also, animals can only obtain K1 from grass and not grains.

MK7 and MK4 are the two subsets of Vitamin K2. MK7 is an essential K2 form, but MK4 has been observed to provide better benefits. It is ideal to take at least 2,000 mcg of K1 and K2 per day, in which 100 mcg of this must be in MK7 form. You can take this at mealtime along with Vitamin D supplement.

Magnesium

Magnesium is an important yet often underappreciated nutrient. This is a crucial ingredient for more than 300 enzyme processes including the production of ATP. This is also essential for proper transcription of RNA and DNA.

Deficiency in magnesium should not be ignored. The symptoms include migraines, nausea, heart arrhythmias, metabolic syndrome, muscle cramps, and tachycardia. This is also linked with PMS, anxiety disorders, asthma, diabetes, and cardiovascular disorders.

Almost everyone must take magnesium supplements. Because of poor farming practices and soil depletion, it is now very difficult to source enough magnesium from food sources alone. Most Americans don't meet the RDA that is already too minimal. The ideal starting dosage is 200 mg per day. This supplement usually comes in different forms: orotate, threonate, glycinate, malate, and citrate. This is best to take before bedtime.

Zinc and Copper

Zinc is an important mineral that enhances mood, boosts energy production, and supports healthy immune function. It is crucial to replenish zinc levels daily because it is difficult to get enough amount of this nutrient from food, and the human body has no capacity for zinc storage.

On the other hand, the human body requires zinc to improve heart and vascular function. Most Americans are deficient in copper, taking only 0.8 mg daily. This is alarming because <1 mg per day can contribute to a higher risk of heart attacks.

Modern dietary practices and farming have caused lower copper intake over the last century. Many fruits, vegetables, and processed meats today don't contain enough copper.

Zinc and copper should be taken together as a supplement because too much zinc can affect the level of copper in the body. As a combo, these supplements can form the body's strongest natural defense mechanism known as copper-zinc superoxide dismutase or CuZnSOD.

This combo supplement is usually in capsule form. The ideal dosage is 1 to 2 mg copper orotate daily and 15 mg zinc orotate daily. Don't take this supplement together with phytates, calcium and iron. These compounds can affect proper zinc absorption.

Iodine

This nutrient is important for metabolism and proper thyroid function. It also helps in the prevention of brain damage and enhancement of immune function. Most Americans are also deficient in iodine, so taking supplements is recommended.

The human body can lose iodine through sweat, so those who are physically active are at particularly high risk for iodine deficiency.

Iodine is mainly sourced from seafood. So you will not get enough of it unless you are eating seafood every day. Don't forget to consult your doctor before taking iodine supplement, especially if you are suffering from a thyroid condition.

The ideal dosage is at least 150 mcg per day. Iodine supplements are usually in potassium iodide capsules or kelp powder. You can take one capsule every day after meals.

L-Tyrosine

Another important supplement that you should take especially if you are into intermittent fasting is the amino acid known as L-Tyrosine. This helps in improving the health of your glands, boosts cognition and mood, and improves response to physical and mental stress.

L-Tyrosine is also proven to easily cross the blood-brain barrier to increase the levels of neurotransmitters norepinephrine, epinephrine, and dopamine. This is also an important building block for thyroid hormone.

While the human body can produce its own L-Tyrosine, it can be depleted because of stress. The ideal dosage for pure L-Tyrosine is at least 500 mg per day. You can take it whenever you want.

Methyl Folate and Methyl B12

Many Americans are deficient in Vitamin B12, which is an important vitamin for cell regeneration, nerve health, proper immune function, and dementia prevention. B12 also protects against atherosclerosis and lowers homocysteine. It is also essential for sustaining reactions of methylation, which prevents cancer and repairs DNA. The brain is one of the most crucial areas for B12.

Deficiency in folate may cause mental symptoms, even though B12 may cause more problems. Both B12 and folate are essential for proper mental function, and lower levels in one can produce a deficiency in the other. However, folate will not rectify deficiency of B12 in the brain.

Folate is also important for the health and proper functioning of the nervous system and the heart. However, you should consult a doctor before taking this supplement because resolving deficiency in B12 without folate could lead to permanent brain damage.

Similarly, high levels of folate without enough B12 may cause neurological conditions. That is why you should take these two supplements together. The ideal dosage is 800mcg of folinic acid (NOT FOLIC ACID) and 5mg of hydroxocobalamin or methylcobalamin. These supplements are usually in form of lozenges and capsules. You can take these supplements daily with food.

Krill Oil

Fish oil is heavily promoted as an important supplement, and there is some truth in this. Enough dosage of high-quality fish oil can enhance muscle growth, improve brain function, and reduce inflammation. However, poor quality or high dosage can harm your health.

Unfortunately, many brands available in local grocery stores are of low potency, oxidized, and contaminated. You are much better off staying away from fish oil if you can't find a high-quality brand.

A better alternative to fish oil is krill oil, which is more stable and easier to use for the brain. It also comes with a strong antioxidant known as astaxanthin.

Krill oil (DHA and EPA) is recommended for those who have deficiency in Omega-3. It is difficult to source Omega-3 from diet alone. The ideal RDA for DHA and EPA is 350 mg for proper brain function.

You can easily achieve this RDA if you are eating wild-caught fish and grass-fed meat several times a day. If not, you should take supplements for at least 500 mg of krill oil every day.

Taking the right forms of supplements is crucial when you are into intermittent fasting. You are cutting down on your diet, so you need to supplement the vitamins and minerals that you should get enough of them.

Be sure to consult your doctor about taking health supplements and mention that you want to try intermittent fasting. Ask for an individualized plan that can work for your health condition and goal.

Spartans Up!

Spartan soldiers were trained to survive on scarcity. Food was rationed, and young initiates were even forced to scavenge and even steal their food. Now, I don't encourage you to steal your supplements. Instead, you should understand the importance of supplementing your deficiencies so you can survive. Fortunately, there are available health supplements today that you can take so you can boost the benefits of intermittent fasting.

11

Tricks and Tips

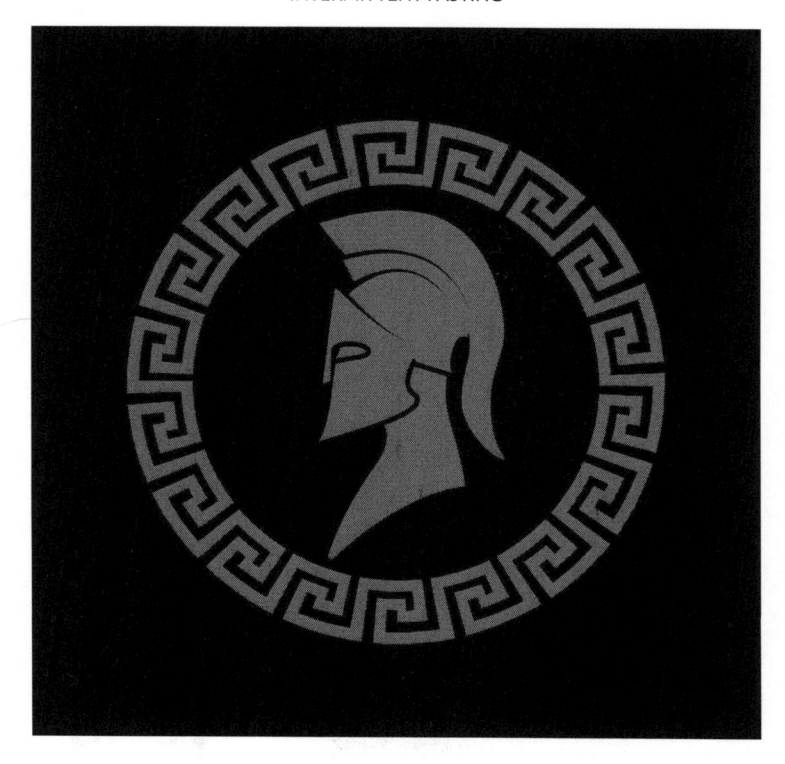

While intermittent fasting has a lot of physical and mental health benefits, you should still be careful as improper practice can also do harm such as becoming dehydrated, losing muscles, and passing out.

To make the most out of intermittent fasting, there are hacks that you can try. In this Chapter, we will discuss some tricks and tips that you can try if you want to try intermittent fasting.

TRICKS AND TIPS

Find Your Why

Intermittent fasting requires passion because you need to stay motivated for an extended period of time. The key to sustain your motivation is to ask yourself why weight loss is important for you.
- Do you want to look better?
- Do you want to feel good about yourself?
- Do you want to be healthier?
- Are you preparing your body for summer?

While you must think beyond the aesthetic reasons, it will help you to list down the things that motivate you so you can be clear on how you can get going. Write down and pin it near your mirror so you can be reminded. Stick to your plan, and during those days that you feel like giving up, just read your list so you can lift up your Spartan spirit again.

Select a Plan that is Suitable to Your Lifestyle

In Chapter 2, we have discussed the different types of intermittent fasting. While Leangains is commonly recommended for beginners, you should choose the plan that is suitable to your lifestyle. You should do this if intermittent fasting is something that you want to adapt for long-term. This may take some time, so be flexible in trying various fasting and feeding windows.

Do Your Research

The fact that you have chosen to read this book and you have reached this Chapter indicates that you are serious in trying intermittent fasting. Aside from this book, you should also read a lot of articles and watch videos online. This will help you learn more about intermittent fasting and cement your decision to pursue it. Why follow something without understanding its benefits? By regularly learning about intermittent fasting you can also share information with your family and friends who may benefit from this diet regimen.

Establish Realistic Goals

Setting up realistic goals is one of the first things you need to do if you want to lose weight through intermittent fasting. This diet regimen is a gradual process to help you lose weight slowly but surely.

Losing half a kilo of body weight is doable and healthy. Leveling up your expectations will also give you more motivation to keep you going. Don't expect too much from this diet regimen because it is impossible to lose 5 kilos in a week. This will only cause disappointment. Goals that are difficult to achieve could be the biggest hurdle you may face. Hence, you should be practical about your expectations.

Establish Short Term Goals

Apart from your ultimate goal, you should also work on your short-term goals. Rather than concentrating too much on losing 10 lbs in six months, you should also figure out how you can achieve this gradually. You can do this by listing down your process goals. This includes counting your calories, setting up your fasting schedule, drafting a meal plan, and other stepping stones towards your ultimate goal. With this, you can experience small bits of successes that will help you keep your motivation.

Be Your Own Coach

Motivation is crucial to be successful with intermittent fasting. However, no one can motivate you well but yourself. The human mind is similar to a computer that you can program so it will exactly think what we tell it to think about. Always remind yourself about your reasons why you are doing this diet regimen and motivate yourself by saying good things about your efforts.

Regularly tell yourself that you can overcome food cravings. You are doing this for your body. Every day, you can program your body and mind to become effective in burning fat. Motivating yourself will enable your brain to believe everything you say so be cautious what you are telling yourself. Whether you think that you will succeed or you will fail, you are right! It all boils down on what you are telling your mind to think about.

Monitor Your Calorie Intake

If weight loss is your goal for trying intermittent fasting, you should definitely count your calories. You may come across some sources of information saying that you can eat whatever you like and you will lose weight as long as you fast for a specific amount of time.

Fasting for several hours can induce calorie deficit, which is crucial for losing weight. However, this is not immediate. Even if you fast for 16 hours, then eat three big meals for the rest of the day, you are possibly consuming the same number of calories.

If you don't monitor your calorie intake, you may end up gaining weight despite fasting for long hours. So make certain that you are counting your calorie intake every day. You can use a food journal or an app. The goal is to create a calorie deficit if you want to lose weight.

One hack you can try to avoid overeating for your first meal is to break your fast with a handful of nuts and a piece of fruit. This can take the edge off your hunger, then you can eat a large meal an hour later. Without the cravings, you can enjoy your meal and stop when you are full.

TRICKS AND TIPS

Be Busy During Fasting Hours

You may feel amazing during your first day of intermittent fasting. You are trying something new and you will love the increased energy and mental clarity you will feel during your fasting window. But the succeeding days could be overwhelming with mixed emotions of sadness, doubt, and cravings for food.

Being busy is the best way to get through this phase. Begin intermittent fasting on a day or a week that you need to do a lot of things. Stay away from doing things that involve food. That is torture. Avoid restaurants, grocery stores, and if possible the kitchen. Stop watching other people preparing food or eating, and don't look for recipes online for your next meal.

Stay Hydrated

Drink at least a glass of water within 30 minutes of waking up. If you feel hungry, drink another glass. Drinking a lot of water during your fasting window will keep your stomach full and will increase your mental alertness.

Avoiding water for a long time can be dangerous because dehydration can result in kidney stones, constipation, mood changes, and unclear thinking.

In general, you should drink 8 to 10 glasses of water, but according to the Centers for Disease Control and Prevention, you just need to drink water whenever you are thirsty.

Stay away from energy drinks even those that are promoted as containing zero calories. Instead, drink tea while fasting because it will not derail the purpose of fasting. Tea should be plain. Don't add milk, cream or sugar.

Coffee is also allowed during the fasting window. But it should be black. Don't add cream, milk or sugar because these will add calories to the drink. Stay away from coffee drinks sold in most coffee shops because they usually contain milk or syrup. Limit your caffeine to only two cups during your fasting window then instead load up on water.

Use Rituals

Using rituals will help you to stay motivated with intermittent fasting because it will help you visualize yourself for success. Some people brush their teeth to signal that they are ready to fast. This particular tip will also help you get rid of food cravings as it will trick the mind that you have already eaten. Other people also perform household chores like cleaning their closet to distract themselves from hunger.

Chew Gum

Chewing sugar-free gum will not derail the purpose of intermittent fasting. This will, in fact, help you while fasting as it satisfies the mouth's need to chew something.

Chewing mint gums can also fight against bad breath that is common during intermittent fasting.

Fight Bad Breath

Once you start intermittent fasting, you will soon discover that one common side effect of this diet is bad breath. This can be embarrassing so you need to fight this one.

The amount of saliva in your mouth can affect the smell of your breath. Saliva is crucial in keeping the pH level and acidity correct in the mouth, which is important to suppress the growth of bacteria that causes stinky breath.

Therefore, if you are not drinking enough water, you will not have enough saliva to do this job. Bacteria will breed in your mouth, and they will ferment food particles left in the mouth. This increases decay and stinky breath.

Drinking a lot of water can combat dry mouth and bad breath. So keep drinking the recommended eight glasses every day, and be sure to floss and brush your teeth and tongue regularly.

Eat Healthy, Delicious Meals

Don't torture yourself by just limiting your diet with salads. One of the advantages of intermittent fasting is that it provides you with more flexibility in your diet to try foods that you might have restricted before. (Just don't overdo with pizza and carbs).

Intermittent fasting allows you to eat bigger meals, so while you are putting limits during your fasting hours, there is no need to limit yourself too much during your feed hours. So don't just eat a small bowl of chef salad and call it a day.

It is fine to enjoy the foods you really love. Enjoy a cookie and don't be afraid to savor a ribeye. You just need to make certain that you are eating enough during your feeding state. This will make sure that you will not be too hungry during your next fasting phase. You should aim to eat healthy 90% of the time, and be sure to include protein and healthy fats.

Get Enough Protein

Make certain that your meals include good sources of protein such as grass-fed chicken. This is essential for satiety and to ensure that you will not lose muscle in the process as discussed in Chapter 6.

Your Meals Should Be Low Glycemic

When eating, ensure that the meals you choose are low-glycemic. This will ensure that your sugar levels are more stabilized every day. Low-glycemic foods include high-fiber whole grains, oats, kale, spinach, and poultry.

Go Easy on the Gym

You may need to go easy on working out in the first two to three weeks of intermittent fasting. You may also need to make some changes to your workout sessions as some cardio exercises can increase your hunger. Another alternative is to change the time that you work out and fit it during your feeding window. Just be patient, because, with time, it will be easier to fit exercise with intermittent fasting.

Take Pictures to Track Your Progress

The scale will not always tell the truth about your progress for weight loss. There is always the possibility of gaining weight when you are building muscle. A good way to keep track of your progress and see the visible results is to take good pictures. Try taking a shot at least once a month. With this, it will be easier to see the proof that this diet is working for you. While your weight will stay the same, you might see that your body will become leaner.

Another way to keep track of your progress is to use available apps so you can see how much time you have fasted to keep tabs of your progress. When you are craving to eat something, just open the app and check how far you have gone so far. Once you are aware that your body usually goes into burning fat between 12 and 16 hours, and you are already in your 13th hours, you can assure yourself that you will eat in a few hours.

You can be motivated if you use a mobile app that will average your weekly fasting. Monitoring your daily averages can be the right motivation you need to do more. Also, checking your app regularly several times daily can be the ideal distraction to stay away from your cravings.

Modify Your Work and Home Environment

Out of sight, out of mind! Ditch your unhealthy snacks from the cupboard and from office desk drawer. And while seeds, whole-grain crackers, and nuts can be nutritious eating them at the wrong time can contribute a lot to your calorie intake. When these snacks are easy to reach, you will definitely give in.

Add Fiber-Rich Fruits and Vegetables

Fruits and vegetables should be added in your everyday meals. The human body takes a bit more time to digest dietary fibers so you will feel fuller for longer.

Fiber is also important while into intermittent fasting because this acts as a buffer to reduce the effects of carbohydrates on blood sugar. It is also crucial in improving the body's sensitivity to insulin.

Fiber also serves as the main factor to maintain a healthy digestive system, and many studies reveal that people who eat more fiber are healthier and live longer. So be sure that your meals include foods that are rich in fiber, especially nuts, whole grains, and vegetables.

Set an Alarm for Eating

There will be instances that you will get caught up in your work or other daily activities that you may even forget to eat during your feeding window. This can happen if you are already into intermittent fasting for several months. While fasting is beneficial to your health, eating when your fasting ends is crucial for your energy levels and overall nutrition.

Get Enough Sleep

Sleep is not only beneficial for your overall health. It is also an important part of your fasting window. You will not feel hungry if you are sleeping. It is ideal to time your sleep to give you a head start.

For instance, if you choose your feeding window in the evening, you can choose to enjoy an early dinner the night before you start your fasting window. When you wake up in the morning, you already spent at least half of your fasting window.

It is also not ideal to begin fasting when you are not sleeping enough. This will make fasting hard.

Forgive Yourself

Intermittent fasting is not easy. There will be instances that you may slip and give in to your cravings. There are times that you have to attend a gathering and while there you were forced to eat instead of fast. This is just normal and humane. But rather than punishing yourself, you must immediately go back on track.

If you have slipped yesterday, make certain that you will stick to your fast today. Don't punish yourself by starving for an extended time. Even Spartan warriors made an error in their judgment.

One of the consequences of being unforgivable to yourself is thinking that intermittent fasting is not effective. This will affect your willpower and will convince you to give up. Be strong and stay away from this trap. This can even result in emotional overeating.

Spartans Up!

As soldiers, Spartans were trained with various tricks to help them achieve their goals. They were trained in stealth, espionage, and other warfare tricks. You can use the tips and tricks discussed in this Chapter to help you overcome the hardships that you will surely experience once you start intermittent fasting.

12

Creating a Spartan Lifestyle of Intermittent Fasting

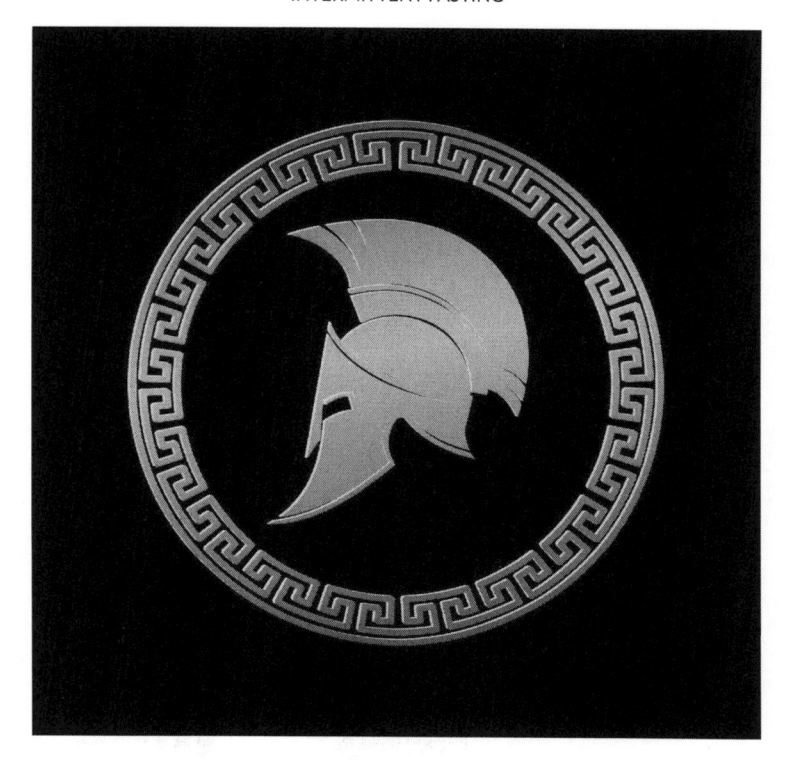

The key to becoming successful in intermittent fasting is to not approach this as a diet but instead of integrating it into your lifestyle like ancient Spartan warriors. Intermittent fasting should not be treated as a health fad, but you should adapt to it as a way of life. Fast. Exercise. Be healthy.

CREATING A SPARTAN LIFESTYLE OF INTERMITTENT FASTING

The Spartan Psyche

Spartan warriors fight just as excellent in the scorching heat and in the pouring rain. They were trained to defeat their enemies regardless of the environment. Like the Spartans, you should treat yourself at war. Your enemies are obesity, disease, and aging.

A bit of precipitation should not let you down. Stress at work? Don't overeat. Get up and hit the gym. You are tired? Everyone can be tired.

If you want to follow the Spartan psyche, you should not be making any excuses. You already know what to do, why should you do it tomorrow? Your ultimate priority should be your well-being and personal health. Stop giving in to your cravings. Stop skipping your workouts.

Spartans can fight their enemies anytime and anywhere! Stuck at home? You can still exercise inside your room. There are many exercises that you can search online that will help you boost the benefits of intermittent fasting.

For Spartans, giving up is not an option. The Spartan army faced the Persian army, which is way bigger then they have ever seen. During the Battle of Thermopylae, the Spartans knew that the army of King Xerxes can end their lives and possibly cause the extinction of Sparta unless they submit to the foreign invader.

However, the Spartan Psyche is so strong that they are well

trained not to surrender. For a Spartan, the highest glory that one can achieve in his life is to die on the battlefield in service of the country. So in spite of guaranteed defeat, the Spartan warriors know only one way: fight!

If you are now out of shape, and you are considering changing this through intermittent fasting, you should definitely follow the Spartan Psyche. Be fearless. Never give up. You should fight!

It is human to feel fear. But it is your choice if you want to submit. If you surrender to fear, it will imprison you and prevent you from living a life that you deserve. You may be overweight now and it may seem impossible to get into shape. But you should tell yourself that you are a child of Sparta, so you should fight!

The results may be slow, but you should move no matter what. One day at a time, one meal at a time.

Fast As If Your Life Depends on It (It's True)

A large part of this book is devoted to the discussion of the health benefits of intermittent fasting. It has high potential to help you live a healthier and longer life.

So fast as if your life depends on it. In fact, this is true. You should treat this lifestyle seriously.

If you are planning to get into intermittent fasting because you want to try a "health fad" then you are still bulking up beyond your calorie count, sorry but you don't mean business.

You are doing it wrong if you are "fasting" then during your feeding hours you eat carbs, sweets, then ignore the need for exercise. You need to think like a Spartan, fast like a Spartan, and prepare like a warrior so that you are ready to fight like one.

You should begin looking at every fasting window like a battle. Take a few minutes to prepare your mindset before you start fasting. Pump your mind into the battle as you visualize winning.

While fasting, get rid of every distraction that can invite you to break the fast early. Do what you need to do. You are a Spartan and you are born to be fit and win battles. It's in your blood.

But this is not to say that you should go kill yourself trying to pursue intermittent fasting. It is your responsibility to give it all whenever you fast. Exert extra effort to explore your capacity. If you can fast for 12 hours, try adding two more hours the next day. See if you can fast for one whole day.

Put yourself in the challenger of channeling your inner Sparta as you start your health journey with intermittent fasting. Think about achieving freedom from the tyranny of fear and from the bondage of being overweight.

As you battle towards winning for health, you become stronger, faster, and better Spartan warrior.

Conclusion

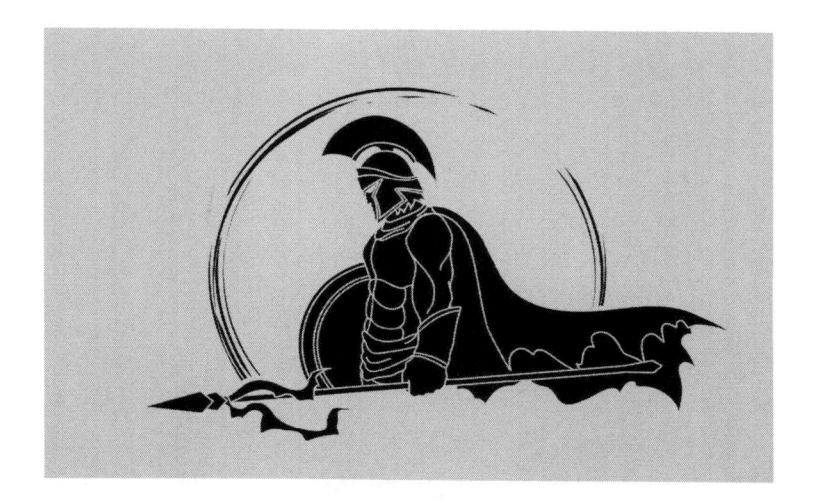

Thank you again for downloading this book!

I hope this beginner's guide to intermittent fasting was able to help you learn the benefits of this ancient diet regimen that is now regaining its ground.

If you are not yet completely convinced that intermittent fasting is suitable for you or skipping breakfast is not suitable for your lifestyle, then it is best to try this for a few weeks and take note

CONCLUSION

of the experience.

The human body has enough glycogen stored in the liver, around 400 calories worth of energy when necessary. This is on top of added fat that you can burn regardless if you are fat or lean. So there is no need to worry that you will die if you don't eat for just a few hours. Even if you decide to fast for days, your body still has enough energy reserves.

Probably you are already convinced that intermittent fasting is the right eating habit for you. Many people are excited to try fasting, but you should not be too reckless about this. You still need to get the opinion of your doctor so you are certain that this can really help you achieve your health goals.

Don't forget to check with your doctor especially if you are managing chronic health conditions or you have a history or has a higher risk of developing eating disorders.

Finally, if you enjoyed this book, then I'd like to ask you for a favor. Would you be kind enough to leave a review for this book on Amazon? It'd be greatly appreciated!

Thank you and good luck!

Disclaimer

This book is not intended as a substitute for the medical advice of physicians. The reader should regularly consult a physician in matters relating to his/her health and particularly with respect to any symptoms that may require diagnosis or medical attention.

Copyright 2018 by Ryan Hunt - All rights reserved.

This document is geared towards providing exact and reliable information in regards to the topic and issue covered. The publication is sold with the idea that the publisher is not required to render accounting, officially permitted, or otherwise, qualified services. If advice is necessary, legal or professional, a practiced

DISCLAIMER

individual in the profession should be ordered.

- From a Declaration of Principles which was accepted and approved equally by a Committee of the American Bar Association and a Committee of Publishers and Associations.

In no way is it legal to reproduce, duplicate, or transmit any part of this document in either electronic means or in printed format. Recording of this publication is strictly prohibited and any storage of this document is not allowed unless with written permission from the publisher. All rights reserved.

The information provided herein is stated to be truthful and consistent, in that any liability, in terms of inattention or otherwise, by any usage or abuse of any policies, processes, or directions contained within is the solitary and utter responsibility of the recipient reader. Under no circumstances will any legal responsibility or blame be held against the publisher for any reparation, damages, or monetary loss due to the information herein, either directly or indirectly.

Respective authors own all copyrights not held by the publisher.

The information herein is offered for informational purposes solely, and is universal as so. The presentation of the information is without contract or any type of guarantee assurance.

The trademarks that are used are without any consent, and the publication of the trademark is without permission or backing by the trademark owner. All trademarks and brands within this book are for clarifying purposes only and are the owned by the owners themselves, not affiliated with this document.

Printed in Great Britain
by Amazon